Your **Personalized Nu**...

Feed Your Skin Right

MARK J. TAGER, MD
Foreword by **DORIS DAY, MD**

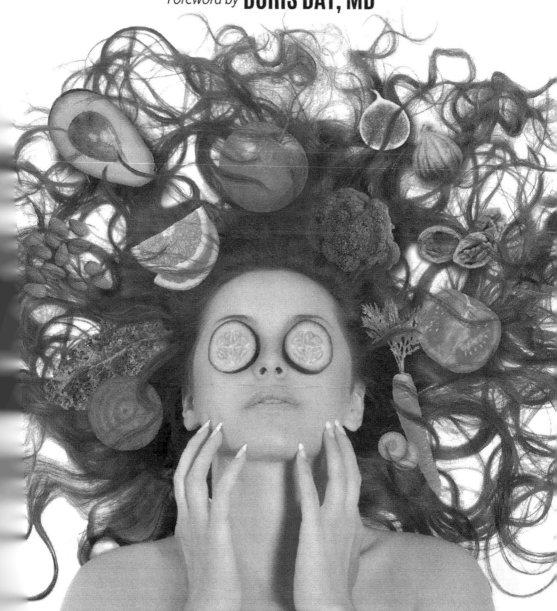

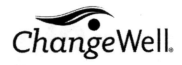

Published in the United States of America by Changewell, Inc.
PO Box 7303
Rancho Santa Fe, CA 92067
www.ChangeWell.com
© 2022 Mark J. Tager, MD

All rights reserved. No part of this publication may be reproduced, stored, or transmitted, in any form or by any method, without express written permission of Changewell, Inc. unless specifically permitted by law, by license, or terms agreed upon with the appropriate reproduction rights organizations. Inquiries regarding reproduction should be addressed to Changewell, Inc. at the address above.

The material contained in this book is not intended to be medical or other professional advice, and should not be considered a substitute for medical or other professional advice. Neither the author nor the publisher is engaged in offering professional advice or services to any individual reader. All matters regarding your health require medical supervision by your own personal physician.

Library of Congress Control Number 2022901462

ISBN: 978-0-9716250-4-4

To order volume copies of *Feed Your Skin Right*, please contact the publisher FYSR@changewell.com

DEDICATION

To H.G. who really does have the baby skin to which we all aspire.

CONTENTS

ACKNOWLEDGEMENTS 7
FOREWORD 11

INTRODUCTION: Your Personalized Nutrition
Prescription for Radiant Beauty.. 13

PART I: What Should I Eat?
Chapter 1: Avoid the Bad Actors for Skin Beauty 29
Chapter 2: Choose This Not That – Making the Most of Your Diet.............. 45
Chapter 3: The Power of Plant Based Eating for Skin Beauty 61
Chapter 4: How Your Gut-Brain-Skin are All Connected 71
Chapter 5: Eating Right for Your Genes 93
Chapter 6: Managing Your Hormones for Skin & Hair Beauty 111
Chapter 7: Lifestyle, Vibrancy, and the Inner Glow 123

PART II: What Supplements Should I Take?
Chapter 8: Setting the Record Straight on Supplements 137
Chapter 9: Vitamins & Minerals for Skin Health & Beauty........................... 149
Chapter 10: Botanicals and Beyond 167
Chapter 11: How to Personalize Your Supplement Regimen 179

PART III: What Topicals Should I Apply?
Chapter 12: Topicals: What Actually Works? 191

PART IV: What Procedures Should I Have?
Chapter 13: Aesthetic Devices, Injectables & Your Skin 217

PART V: Your Personal Plan
Chapter 14: What's *Right* for You... 231

Appendix A – RDAs for Essential Nutrients 241
Appendix B – Micronutrient Deficiencies and Excessive Intakes 247
Appendix C – Common Genetic Variants & Skin Health 255
Bibliography 257
Index 273
About the Author... 285

ACKNOWLEDGEMENTS

There are those moments—for me in the hours before dawn—when two sounds predominate. One of these is external; the clicking sound of fingers contacting computer keys. The other is internal. It is the voices of dozens of researchers, clinicians, teachers, and scientists schooling me on various aspects of aesthetics and nutritional medicine. The result—this book—is a compilation of ideas and recommendations that was created by my inner gang of advisors. My fingers just did the heavy lifting. It is their words that leapt to the pages.

I intensely follow the functional medicine pioneering work of David Perlmutter, MD; Dale Bredesen, MD; Marvin Singh, MD; Joel Evans, MD; Filomena Trindade, MD; Lara Zakaria, PharmD; Sherry Torkos, RPh; Tieraona Low Dog, MD; Patrick Hanaway, MD; Mark Menoloscino, MD; Felice Gersh, MD; Jeff Bland, PhD; Jill Carnahan, MD; Suzanne Gilberg-Lenz, MD; Liz Lipski, PhD; Andrew Heyman MD; Brie Wieselman, LAc; James LaValle, RPh; Mark Hyman, MD; Stacie Stephenson, DC; and Frank Lipman, MD. Their voices resonate so strongly in my brain, I can't tell where their thoughts end and mine begin. I am thankful, however, that they've taken up residence in my cranium. If you are not following these docs on social media, I highly encourage you to do so.

There are always friends and colleagues who volunteer to read over manuscripts and provide feedback. Then there are the ones that really take the time to diligently make corrections and suggestions. Enrique Jacome, MD, Isabella Davis, and Michelle Le Beau are in this small but powerful group. Heartfelt thanks to my four favorite naturopathic physicians Peter Bongiorno, ND, LAc; Adam Silberman, ND; Alex Keller, ND; and Kendra Etzel, ND; who slogged through the text to make certain I got most things right, and what I didn't is my fault alone. And a big shout out to Jessica Titchenal, DCN, one of the bright lights in the field on personalized nutrition who also read over every word of this book (my heroine!) as did one of my favorite Integrative docs, Hetal Patel, MD.

Ever since I got involved in the aesthetic world in 2001, I've been blessed to know practitioners who combine an eye for beauty with a bright mind and skilled hands. In the words of the old Billy Crystal skit on Saturday Night Live, they each look MAHVELOUS, and they help their patients look marvelous as well. You'll find tips and hints from a dozen or so of my favorite dermatologists and skin specialists in the text. These are some of my closest "buds" in the biz: Heidi Waldorf, MD; Suneel Chilukuri, MD; Michelle Henry, MD; Sonia Badreshia-Bansal, MD (along with her plastic surgeon husband Vivek Bansal, MD); Terrence Keaney, MD; Vic Ross, MD; Reena Jogi, MD; Claudia Hernandez, MD; Jorge Krasovsky, MD; Glynis Ablon, MD; and Lori Robertson, FNP-C. These clinicians are each as beautiful on the inside as they are on the outside; however, none being more attractive, in my eyes, than Doris Day, MD, who graciously contributed the Foreword.

For those of you who knew Dr. Richard Fitzpatrick, you'd understand why my eyes always tear up in his memory. He gave so much to so many. He's a permanent resident in my heart, and I always take a moment to honor him whenever I write about aesthetics.

In the course of writing, it's all too common to get stuck. The fix is usually a dose of creativity. For this moment of inspiration, I will occasionally step back and ask WWSD? What would Steve do? Although he knows more about how to sculpt beauty than to infuse it nutritionally, I am always inspired by the most creative mind in the aesthetics field: Facial Plastic Surgeon Steven Dayan, MD. I've had the honor of working with him on the Miami Cosmetic Surgery meeting.

Many thanks to those who helped me get the words *right*. (As you'll see RIGHT is a BIG part of this book.) This includes my colleagues at The American Nutrition Association (theana.org): Dana Reed, MSNc; Corrine Bush, CNS; Victoria Yunez Behm, CNS; Jackie Chiuchiarelli; and Mike Stroka, JD, CNS, who is guiding the ANA's ship through some wonderful sailing waters.

A book about aesthetics must be pretty. To this end, I can't thank the Enzymedica team enough, especially Bob Jankowski as he patiently worked through multiple editions of the cover. Scott Sensenbrenner, CEO of Enzymedica, Julia Craven, and Michelle Le Beau kept me consumer-focused throughout the process. My business partners, Robert John Hughes and Indira Hodzic provided ongoing encouragement. I've always been impressed with how Mei Wei Wong (graphics) and Karen Edwards (words) help me sort through and organize my midnight ramblings. Karen did way too much research for this book, enough to do another five at least. She was aided editorially by my son James, who is a word-guy par excellence and a powerful writer/editor. When's he's not "on a righteous quest for justice," he always gifts his time to me to refine my narrative.

Every book needs friends and family who can provide a reality check to see if the content resonates. I'm honored to have Anastasia Zadeik head this team. She had me trim some fat, as well as add some muscle to the text.

As this is my 11th book, I've given big shout outs in earlier works to my parents, wife, and kids. I'm down to the two newest additions to my spiritual cohort: Sienna, my 10-year-old Maltipoo who was by my side for 80% of the writing, and our first granddaughter Harper, who was responsible—lovingly—for 80% of the delightful distractions.

Heartfelt gratitude to you all.

FOREWORD

Doris Day, MD

His LinkedIn profile seems to sum it up:

Healthcare Synergist/Medical Messaging Maven/Speaker/Author.

Having had the pleasure of knowing and working with Dr. Mark Tager for more than a decade, he fits these descriptors, and more.

One of the dictionary definitions of "synergist" is quite succinct. A synergist is "An agent that participates in an effect of synergy." Synergy instills new possibilities in people. There are few people in the health and aesthetic industries who do this better than Mark.

Mark confided to me that early on, he realized he had a gift that he could bestow unto others above and beyond taking care of patients one-to-one. He recognized that his skills were best suited for communicating one-to-many. Within the field of health and beauty, he mastered the media—print, audio, video, and online communication skills that he often teaches other healthcare professions. In the fields of aesthetics and integrative medicine, he is well known for helping practitioners become "irresistibly powerful communicators."

Perhaps the reason we're on the same wavelength is that I too, share the passion for communication: not just sharing knowledge, but also translating complicated science into easy to understand and actionable bites. Trained as a journalist and medical reporter before becoming a physician, I value the power and importance of educating both my patients and the public, as well as my peers. I'm always happy to treat the patient in front of me but I'm just as happy to reach a larger audience when I can.

These communication skills are important because there is so much misinformation about skin care and beauty in the market. It is refreshing to have clear voices providing accurate information that is easy to follow and understand. Today, with the explosion of digital technology, communication comes in so many forms. With so many ways to access information, there is still nothing that replaces the pages of a book that can be felt, read and re-read, highlighted, and saved for later review. This medium is timeless and will always be my favorite way to communicate and learn.

Having practiced dermatology for more than 20 years, I've noticed some things stay the same, and others change. Yes, everyone wants their skin to glow, their spots to vanish, and their wrinkles and folds to disappear, or at least be artfully minimized. But so many of today's patients are wanting more. They are increasingly asking about diet, supplements, genetics, the microbiome, and skin allergies. The same young person who comes into my office for "prejuvenation"—treatment to get ahead of skin aging—will ask what else they can do to increase and retain their beauty. Invariably the discussion will turn to "skin inside." Here's where I'll make the easiest referral, and that's to the wisdom and practical information in *Feed Your Skin Right*.

There's another definition of "synergist" that I like. A synergist is someone in a group or team who sets their personal interests below the best interests of the enterprise as a whole. With *Feed Your Skin Right,* Mark is once again raising the bar and the industry as a whole.

Introduction

YOUR PERSONALIZED NUTRITION PRESCRIPTION FOR RADIANT BEAUTY

You may have been drawn to this book for the promise of radiant, glowing, beautiful skin, or perhaps because you are a passionate student of nutrition and natural approaches to wellness. Maybe you are seeing the signs of accelerated aging and wonder what other self-care measures you can take.

When it comes to beauty, my educated guess is that right now you're doing half the work. You see a skincare specialist whose anti-aging treatments include light-based therapies, radio-frequency, cryotherapy, or needling. You periodically get facials or peels. You are not unacquainted with neurotoxins or fillers, or even surgery for that matter. You regularly use sunblock to protect your skin from UVA/UVB damage. And, your bathroom cabinet contains at least a half-dozen of the latest, greatest cosmeceuticals, all in different states of use or disuse.

Regular skincare, sun protection, periodic professional and technology-assisted refreshing—these all produce results, but they are part of the equation, not the entire solution. There's an equally important part that many of us don't consider.

As you sit here reading this book, 15% of your blood flow is going through your skin. Each day your heart beats about 100,000 times, pumping 6 liters of blood throughout the body. Your bloodstream supplies oxygen, amino acids, carbohydrates, fats, minerals, vitamins, antioxidants, and other key co-factors to the skin. These are key elements for both skin health and beauty. The bloodstream also removes the waste products and toxins from the skin.

What you put in your mouth—your diet and intelligent supplementation—provides your skin with what it needs from the *inside out*. This inside-out approach to skin health, coupled with regular skin care, is what results in radiant beauty, the glow that emits from skin that optimally reflects light.

THE RIGHT APPROACH

The most important word in the book's title is the word *RIGHT*, what's right for YOU. There are 7 billion people on the planet, and no two have the exact same combination of lifestyle habits, genetics, microbiome, environmental exposure, medical history, supplement or medication use, not even identical twins. Put simply, there is no other person on the planet with skin identical to yours. There is just one YOU, something that researchers who deal with numbers in scientific studies call the "N of 1." If you want to create skin health and beauty from the inside out, you'll need to do what's best for you, not someone else.

This book details the evolution of a health and wellness field called *personalized nutrition*. In years past, personalized nutrition was a mere few steps beyond the original, generic one-size-fits-all diets recommended to patients for weight loss or cardiovascular health. Today, we have the tools at our disposal to better tailor individual treatments for people who want skin health and beauty.

Explosions in our understanding of genetics are shedding light on the individual variations that lead to premature wrinkling, loss of facial volume, dehydration, excessive pigmentation, and conditions such as rosacea and eczema. The technology to rapidly and cost-effectively examine some, or all, of the human genome can help guide us to "eat right for our genes." Our deepening understanding of nutrigenomics can explain why a certain diet can be right for one person but wrong for another. Nutrigenomics can also reveal health conditions you are at risk for, and why you may need additional nutritional supplementation to obtain optimal balance and prevent specific insufficiencies.

The skin is your body's largest organ and the first line of defense between you and the outside world. If you feed it right—on the inside and on the outside—it will not only perform its job, but you will remain vibrant and youthful looking.

In the last few decades, researchers have begun to unravel the powerful connections that the GI microbiome—the 100 trillion bacteria, fungi, and viruses that inhabit your gut—play in communicating both positively and negatively with your brain and skin. While research is lagging behind with respect to the gut microbiome, many of the largest cosmeceutical companies are pouring money into understanding the skin microbiome and its contribution to health and beauty. Like the gut, each region of the skin has its own unique flora, and upsets in bacterial diversity and quality contribute to many common skin conditions. You'll learn a lot more about the skin microbiome and the gut-brain-skin axis as we move ahead. While this isn't a book on medical dermatology, I will point out the connection between nutrition, gut health and some of the most common dermatological conditions.

There are also easier-to-understand, science-based recommendations that provide many health and beauty benefits: simple things like slowing down when you eat, expressing gratitude for nourishment, and limiting the time during which you consume calories. This last approach is alternately known as chrononutrition, time restricted eating, or intermittent fasting.

You just can't shovel food into your system all day and night and expect your body to process that food optimally. And when the food is calorically dense, and nutritionally poor, it can contribute to the growing epidemic of insulin resistance. Research has shown that restricting eating to an 8 to 10 hour span during the day can lower elevated insulin levels, improve fat burning, aid in cellular repair, and even change the expression of several genes and molecules related to longevity and disease protection.[1,2] We'll cover the nuances of all this—such as how long and how often to incorporate these approaches into your life—as this book progresses.

CREATING HEALTHIER RELATIONSHIPS

You have relationships with different foods, and just as in life, some relationships may not bring out your best. When it comes to diet, food sensitivities definitely qualify as negative relationships. Certain foods may cause food-related reactions ranging from GI upset to allergies. These allergies often manifest in the skin as rashes, hives, or wheals when we eat certain foods. Depending upon the nature of the allergy, reactions can be near-term, or they can be delayed. Or, in, the case of serious allergic responses, such as anaphylaxis, food allergies can be life threatening. We now have better tests to detect food sensitivities, allergies, and a broad spectrum of other, less damaging but still negative, reactions. In addition, there are even foods that just don't taste good to us, based on genes that control how our tongue detects sweet, sour, salty, bitter and savory tastes.

Dealing with problematic foods today goes beyond simply avoiding the top offenders—milk, eggs, wheat, soy, shellfish, tree nuts, peanuts, fish, and sesame. You also need to try to avoid the chemicals that have been applied to foods not normally considered allergenic. Any number of pesticides (an herbicide like glyphosate/Roundup® is technically a pesticide) can be applied to crops, and even "organic" crops can be affected by aerial drift of these toxins. Pesticides are ubiquitous in the United States, but everyone's exposure is unique: a phenomenon known as toxic load.

Your best defense is to limit your pesticide exposure as much as possible by eating clean (organic) food whenever possible. The nonprofit Environmental Working Group (EWG) puts out its annual "Dirty Dozen" list of fruits and vegetables with the highest pesticide contamination.[3] More recently, EWG developed a "Clean Fifteen" list of produce with the least amount of pesticides to help consumers make better choices. You'll find their recommendations later in the text.

When it comes to cosmetics and personal care products, EWG has identified a bevy of toxic chemicals, some of which act as endocrine disruptors, including parabens and phthalates.[4] These products can also be contaminated with heavy metals such as lead, mercury, arsenic, cadmium, and nickel. These toxins aren't just bad for the people who use them—compromising people's immune function and increasing cancer risk—but also pose a great risk to a pregnant woman when her baby's organs and nervous system are developing.

All the organic eating in the world won't offset the toxicity of personal care products that have become ubiquitous in Americans' daily lives. According to EWG, women use an average of 12 products daily—containing 168 different chemicals—and men use an average of 6 products daily—containing 85 different chemicals. Scarier still, the average teenager uses 17 products, and all of these usage statistics are likely to be on the conservative side. Whether it's soap, shampoo, deodorant, hair coloring, moisturizer or make-up, their ingredients are being absorbed directly into the bloodstream via the body's largest organ—your skin.

Many of us take multiple prescription medications that deplete nutrients from our bodies. That means that no matter how "clean" we eat, we're still losing out. The top 10 drug categories that can lead to nutrient deficiencies include those designed to treat high cholesterol, type 2 diabetes, high blood pressure, acid reflux and heartburn, constipation,

> ### INNER VERSUS OUTER SKIN
>
> In *FYSR*, we'll discuss two types of skin: "outside skin" (the covering of your body) and "inside skin" (your gut lining). You'll learn what each is comprised of; how they work as barrier organs; how they are affected by what you eat; and how they are closely related to each other. The "inside skin" of the gut lining is ever so delicate—just one cell thick—tasked with keeping all the microbes and waste products in the gut, right where they should be—especially if we want great "outside skin." And like the "inside skin," the "outside skin" requires proper nutrition so you can look your best.

depression, bacterial infections (antibiotics), pain, osteoporosis, and drugs to prevent pregnancy (birth control).

ARE YOU READY FOR CHANGE?

There is a time in many people's lives when a light turns on. They get it. They make the connection between what they eat and how they feel, think, and look. This epiphany changes their life for the better. For me, the light turned on when I was in the beginning of my second year at Duke Medical School.

It was a particularly stressful time. Unlike many other medical schools, Duke compressed the first two years of preclinical medical education into one. So, at the beginning of our second year, medical students were thrust into clinical work.

There's a syndrome that affects almost every young medical student. It's fueled by endless reading about diseases and the rote memorization of countless signs and symptoms. This repetitive reinforcement results in the Medical Student Disease: the belief that you've got every single ailment that you've ever studied; whether it is an exotic condition like tsutsugamushi disease or the more common symptoms of a GI ulcer.

So, when I noticed that my skin and the whites of my eyes were appearing a bit more yellow, coupled with a loss of taste for cigarettes (yes, I smoked back in those days), I shrugged it off to reading too much about liver disease. It was only when I noticed my urine turn the color of a cola drink, that it hit me. I had hepatitis. Fortunately, it was the infective kind (fortunate because this was less severe). With rest, the Duke Medicine doctors assured me I would be okay.

Still, it gave me *pause*—one of my favorite words—time to step back and reflect on how my lifestyle was affecting my health and why my skin was yellow, wizened, and itchy. I had aged a decade in just a week. I reflected on my diet of sugary soft drinks and pockets of candies to keep my energy up; my reliance on heavily processed foods; meals eaten while standing; food wolfed down in minutes, if not seconds. Today we know many of these components as the SAD—or Standard American Diet. It's not just slowly killing many Americans; it's also contributing to how we look and feel. The SAD diet was starting to get to me as well.

So, my journey began. I became a vegetarian; now, I'm a pescatarian. I took up jogging, yoga, and meditation. I started playing my guitar again. In short, I made the kind of changes that, for decades, I've advocated to patients and consumers in general.

Along with noted Duke University biochemist Henry Kamin, PhD, I researched nutrition and contributed to one of the first elective courses in nutrition for medical students. In those days, we didn't know that much about the science of nutrition. The concept of personalized nutrition wasn't even on the radar. Still, given the crucial importance of nutrition as both prevention and treatment of so many diseases, it's hard to believe that today's med students, interns, and residents can go through their entire training with little to no education in this basic treatment modality.

In fact, the most recent data (2012) shows that the average medical doctor receives only 19.0 hours of nutrition instruction over 4 years of training, despite the minimum recommendation of 25 hours.[5] (And that minimum recommendation is not a lot better!) This reflects a dismal dip from an average 22.3 hours in 2004, and only slightly less than the average in 2008 (19.5 hours). Less than a third of medical schools in 2012 actually met the guidelines set by the National Academy of Sciences.

Sadly, the medical students want more nutrition training—they're just not getting it—and it's their future patients who will lose out. Nutrition is a root cause in many chronic diseases, such as diabetes, hypertension, and heart disease. If doctors lack nutrition knowledge, they cannot use it as a noninvasive tool to manage a patient's disease, which often leads to poor outcomes for the patient.

Fortunately, there is an entire universe of trained nutrition professionals who can step in and fill this void. The top echelon includes naturopathic doctors (ND), Certified Nutrition Specialists (CNS), and Certified Clinical Nutritionists (CCN). Other clinicians may also have advanced training and experience in personalized nutrition including pharmacists, dentists, registered dieticians and chiropractors. Some health coaches may also have undergone advanced training, although legally they cannot practice medical nutrition therapy.[6] In PART V: Your Personal Plan, I'll point to some resources for identifying professionals who can help guide you.

WHAT LIES AHEAD

At this point, I hope you are intrigued by the promise of radiant skin and enticed by the possibilities of an inside skin beauty approach. I know that attention spans are short, generally speaking, so for those of you who want the "Cliff Notes" summary of what to do, here it is.

THE TAGER TOP TEN FOR SKIN HEALTH & BEAUTY FROM WITHIN

1. **Get Real.** This is the primary message of *FYSR*. Real people eat real food and your skin prefers real food to get the nutrients it needs. By choosing processed foods and fake foods, you sacrifice both health and beauty. Resist the temptation to skip ahead to the supplement recommendations, especially if you have a crappy diet. Supplements alone won't provide you with radiant beauty—you need to accept that fact right from the beginning.

2. **Stop Inflammaging.** Too many Americans are carrying a large inflammatory organ (visceral fat) which oozes reactive compounds into the bloodstream and disrupts satiety signals. Eating an inflammatory diet high in sugars, bad fats, and toxic chemicals promotes fat accumulation around the vital abdominal organs. Inflammation is public enemy number one—and for good reason: it does a lot of damage to the human body. People who follow an anti-inflammatory diet, such as the Mediterranean diet, are some of the healthiest people by far.

    Sugar is a big contributor to inflammation, and the average American eats roughly 100 pounds of simple, refined sugar every year. Sugar is even more insidious when it comes to skin health. Glycation occurs when important proteins, such as collagen, get bound up with the sugar which, in turn, changes both their structure and function in the body. Glycated collagen is a recipe for wrinkles. Consuming more sugar leads to more glycation and more wrinkles. What a great incentive to cut back on sugar!

3. **Plug the Leaks (gut and skin).** A strong barrier function is paramount to your inside and outside skin. The inside skin of the GI tract forms the basis of the gut-brain-skin axis by keeping GI sewage from leaking into the bloodstream. Leaky gut and leaky skin cause undesirable and harmful inflammation within the body and delicate skin layers. We'll go over the 3R approach to strengthening your gut and skin defenses. **R**emove the irritants. **R**epair the barrier. **R**eplace & repopulate the microbiome. Good gut health keeps inflammation in check and strengthens the gut-brain-skin axis. A happy gut equals a happy brain equals happy (and beautiful) skin.

4. **Feed Your Bugs Well.** The 100 trillion microbes in your gut are working for you—more so than we ever knew before—from vitamin synthesis to neurotransmitter and hormone production. The inextricable connections between the gut, brain, and skin require top-notch nutrition, especially if you want glowing skin and a finely-tuned body and mind. You'll learn how to take good care of your gut bugs so they'll take care of you.

5. **Protect the Skin from Within.** Plant-based foods provide 5,000+ phytonutrients, including an abundance of free-radical fighting antioxidants. Mother Nature's rainbow-colored fruits and vegetables contain substances that protect them from environmental stress, and we benefit by consuming them—their nutrients and fiber feed and support our gut bacteria and also help shield our skin from ultraviolet damage. You'll learn just which macronutrients and micronutrients to focus on for optimal skin health.

6. **Eat Right for Your Genes.** Genetic variants play a role in skin health by influencing food preferences, determining nutrient absorption, and predisposing you to increased glycation, wrinkles, decreased skin elasticity, and increased facial pigmentation. Nutrigenomic testing is the future of personalized nutrition—knowing your genetic

predisposition allows you to make positive changes. I'll walk you through the science of this cutting-edge analysis and provide recommendations on the available tests, many of which you can obtain directly online.

7. **Supplement Intelligently.** The operative word is *intelligently*. Begin by making plants the foundation of your diet. Eat the rainbow, but also recognize where you may experience gaps in the protection nutrients afford you due to age, chronic health conditions, genetic predispositions, drug-induced nutrient depletions, environmental toxins, or unhealthy lifestyle. I'll help you understand what constitutes a quality supplement, and why some are better than others. You'll also learn how certain drugs interact with nutrients.

8. **Energize Your Skin**. Mitochondria are the workhorses of the body, responsible for producing the energy our 37 trillion cells need to function efficiently. As we age, these cellular powerhouses decrease in number and power-generating capacity. When this happens in the skin, the deleterious signs of aging creep in. You'll learn the key strategies to keep your mitochondria humming and your skin glowing with the vibrance of your youth.

9. **Time Your Eating**. *When* you eat (and don't eat) is just as important as *what* you eat. Various types of fasting—even while you sleep—allow your cells to achieve a state of autophagy. Think of autophagy like "cellular housekeeping" that cleans up the waste products, such as damaged mitochondria, and recycles them into new functional components for the cells. You'll learn ways to maximize autophagy for rejuvenating worn out skin cells. A good night's sleep is a terrific place to start!

10. **Move It to Max It & Sleep Well**. When it comes to ensuring your skin looks its very best, exercise is often overlooked. But blood flow isn't the only reason exercise is so important. From minimizing glycation to promoting microbial diversity to ensuring mitochondrial health, exercise is an all-around strategy for skin health. If you're a passionate exerciser, you'll enjoy learning about some of the latest science on the skin-beauty connection. If you're more sedentary and looking for new

motivation, perhaps the promise of glowing skin and a good night's rest can get you back into the exercise habit. Restorative sleep does wonders for your entire body.

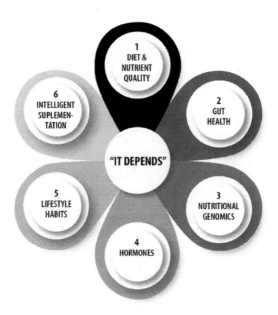

THE FOUR QUESTIONS

As a physician who has spent half of his career in integrative medicine and the other half in aesthetics, I routinely get asked four questions from friends, family members, and interested consumers:

- What should I eat?
- What supplements should I take?
- What topicals should I apply?
- What procedures should I have?

Most people want a single, clear, definitive answer to each of these questions. There is one answer to each, but most people don't like it. *"It depends."* What's right for you depends on the many factors we will be discussing in the pages ahead. The majority of *FYSR* is directed toward skin health and beauty from the inside out—what you should and should not put into your mouth. The "It Depends" wheel above visually organizes the variables that address the first question: What should I eat?

WHAT SUPPLEMENTS SHOULD I TAKE?

The Centers for Disease Control and Prevention (CDC) estimates that anywhere from 57.6-80.2% of Americans take supplements, with the highest use in women over age 60.[7] The most common are multivitamin-mineral supplements, followed by vitamin D, and omega-3 fatty acids. The entire $150B business category of supplements has been given a huge lift in the wake of COVID-19, as consumers move to increase the intake of nutrients that have immune supporting properties, such as vitamin D, echinacea, vitamin C and others. For those who are inclined to more scientifically detailed readings, the American Nutrition Association (theana.org) and the Institute for Functional Medicine (ifm.org) both have excellent position papers on the contribution that supplements can make to immune function.[8,9,10]

In *FYSR*, we'll turn our attention to the supplement category that is actually experiencing one of the fastest growth rates. According to the Nutrition Business Journal, the supplement category "Skin Inside" experienced 9.9% growth in 2021. It is now estimated to be a $1.5B category. The B vitamins, including biotin, make up the largest share of the market, accounting for just over 40% of sales. The greatest growth was fueled in large part by increasing demand for collagen, which went from 8% of the beauty market to the second single largest ingredient and 17.5% market share.[11]

With the increasing number of skin-inside ingredients and products comes growing confusion. Step into any supermarket, specialty nutrition store, or pharmacy, and you will find rows of supplements, all being gazed at by consumers with quizzical looks. What supplements should you take? Again, it depends. However, by the time you get to PART II, you will have already learned the "It Depends" factors from the wheel in PART I, so you'll be well on your way to a deeper personal understanding. I'll clarify how to identify safe, effective supplements. We'll go over the major skin beauty ingredients, how they work, and in which formulations they can be found.

WHAT TOPICALS SHOULD I APPLY?

Shmears are Not Just for Bagels

Topical skincare/beauty is a $135B business, and with tens of thousands of choices, it's confusing. We all want to know, "What should I apply to my skin?" Topical nutrition should complement internal nutrition for enhanced beauty and environmental protection. Some of the very same micronutrients and botanicals we take as dietary supplements have popped up in skin creams, serums, and facial tonics. They hydrate, moisturize, and protect against the sun. I'll explain the rationale for some of the most common bioactive compounds, vitamins, minerals, and probiotics currently being added to the topicals. While I will wade in on my skincare regimen (I'm a guy and it's pretty simple), I've reached out to a handful of the world's leading dermatologists and asked them point-blank: what works, why and how, and if my reader wants to spend hard earned dollars on topicals, which provide the best bang for the dollar? You'll find their recommendations in PART III: What Topicals Should I Apply?

WHAT PROCEDURES SHOULD I HAVE?

Understanding the Magic of More Aggressive Therapies

As part of the team that created the Fraxel® laser, a device that revolutionized skin resurfacing, I've spent many years getting to understand how energy devices affect the skin. Depending on the energy source, these devices stimulate the inner workings of the skin to create more long-lasting beauty. Some of the injectable fillers work in a similar fashion. You'll find my thoughts on how to select the procedure that's right for you. Again, I've leaned on the expertise of several of my colleagues who have more hands-on experience with these types of treatments.

For both nutritional and aesthetic products, you'll find selected product recommendations in the text. My apologies in advance—with thousands of products coming to market every year, I know what I know *today*. Tomorrow will surely be different. My colleagues and I are also biased in our selections. We know, and recommend, those products for which we have personal experience. Just to put your mind at rest, I receive no compensation from any supplement sales.

Embarking on Your Journey

I trust I've got you excited about your journey toward radiant beauty. Before embarking, I'll leave you with a question that I've pondered for some time. I suppose it has some philosophical undertones. *Is it possible to have a really crappy diet and beautiful skin?*

The answer is "possible, but not likely." If you're young and healthy, with an amazing metabolism, a powerful immune system, and you get lots of physical activity…well, just maybe you can cheat time. You may be able to get by for a while, but poor nutrition eventually catches up with you. So, let's flip the question: *If you want to have glowing, radiant skin, do you need to pay attention to your diet?* The answer is absolutely "yes," and every day, science continues to affirm this.

Part One:
What Should I Eat?

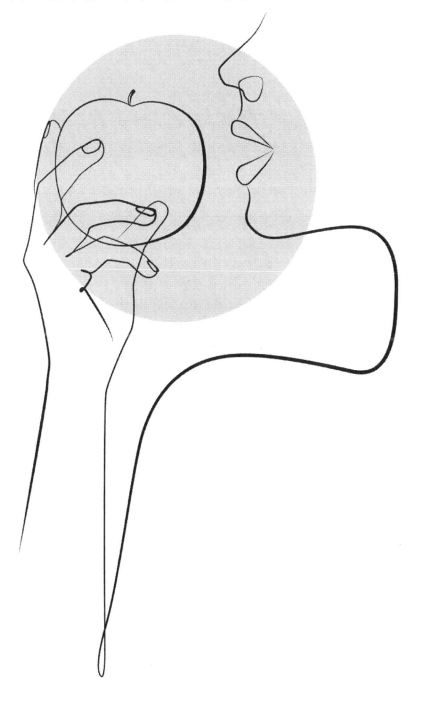

"To eat is a necessity, but to eat intelligently is an art."

Francois de la Rochefoucauld

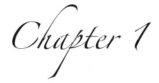

Chapter 1

AVOID THE BAD ACTORS FOR SKIN BEAUTY

In the Introduction I addressed the question of "What should I (you) eat? by providing two essential, yet confounding words of guidance.

It depends.

First of all, it depends on the extent to which you are SAD, in other words, consuming the Standard American Diet. This is a diet that is high in refined carbohydrates, deficient in fiber, and low in vitamins, minerals, and good essential fatty acids. For many Americans, it is too much nutrient-poor food, consumed too quickly, with too little forethought, preparation, and appreciation. It's a diet that's contributed to 42.4% of adults being obese, 47% hypertensive, and 10.5% diabetic.[12,13,14] These nutrition-related conditions savagely cut years off our lives while contributing to more disability and lower quality of life. They also don't help our skin be at its best. Let's look more closely at the culprits causing unhealthy skin.

When It Comes to Sweetness, We're Number 1!
Americans are number one when it comes to sugar consumption, with an astounding 126.4 grams per day according to Euromonitor and WorldAtlas.[15,16] In more relatable terms, that's one-quarter of a pound, and in dramatic, rather scary terms, that's like eating through a 5-pound bag of sugar every 3 weeks, or nearly 90 pounds for the year. Pew Research—more favorably—suggested that America's sweet tooth peaked in 1999 and has been on the decline since (77 pounds in 2014).[17] Certainly, the data are lagging and have yet to factor in any influence due to the COVID-19 pandemic (such as stress/sweets eating). The World Health Organization recommends eating no more than 25 grams of sugar daily,

so we are 3-4 times (300%-400%) over our limit. Without a doubt, we're eating a whole lot more sugar than 200 years ago when we only ate about 2 pounds of sugar annually.

Even since the 1970s, the *type* of sugar consumed has changed, from mostly refined cane and beet sugars to corn sugars. Compounding the problem are hidden sugars added to processed foods that you would not expect to be in there, in quantities that do little other than promote America's sweet tooth. Even foods that are considered "healthy" often contain inordinate amounts of simple carbohydrates and "hidden" sugars.

EVERYDAY PRODUCTS WITH HIDDEN SUGAR

- Breakfast cereals
- Instant oatmeal
- Yogurt
- Granola/protein bars
- Nut butters
- Smoothies
- Dried fruit
- Pasta sauces
- Salad dressings
- Ketchup/BBQ sauce/other condiments

SUGAR AND YOUR SKIN

While there are multiple factors that contribute to obesity, from the standpoint of skin beauty, this turn toward sugar creates its own unique biochemical complication: *glycation*. Glycation is the binding of a glucose or fructose molecule to an essential protein or lipid. This changes the molecular structure. As a result of this binding, so-called rogue molecules called advanced glycation end products (AGEs) are generated. AGEs are associated with increased oxidative damage and implicated in some diseases, in aging, and in the micro and macrovascular complications in diabetes.

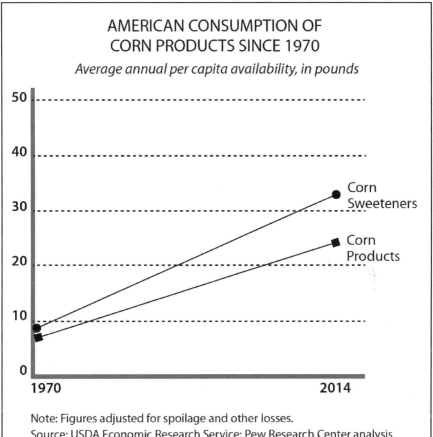

COOKING TECHNIQUES TO REDUCE AGEs IN YOUR DIET
- Cook at lower temperatures for shorter durations.
- Use a slow cooker on low heat.
- Cook meats with moist heat (steam, stew, poach & braise).
- Avoid grilling, roasting, broiling or frying meats.
- Marinate meats with acidic ingredients (i.e., lemon juice or vinegar).
- Cook sous vide (water bath for extended time).

Changing your eating habits—or at least the way you cook your animal-based foods—will lower the amount of AGEs generated. Cooking from scratch with whole and minimally processed foods puts you in control and is a surefire way to avoid the AGEs in heavily processed foods.

Glycation affects the skin by inducing wrinkles to form. Glycated collagen becomes rigid and the skin begins losing its flexibility and suppleness. Unlike everyday, garden-variety fine lines and wrinkles, which are linear in appearance and run parallel to each other, the wrinkles due to glycation have a distinct cross-hatched appearance. Imagine a 50-year-old lifelong smoker who has a face of someone who looks 120. These wrinkles are what we'd consider deep, unattractive, and premature. Glycation may also contribute to thinning of the skin and discoloration.

Glycated collagen doesn't just suddenly occur when you first notice fine lines or wrinkles; for most people, the visible signs begin around age 35. Glycated collagen can in fact, be scientifically first observed at age 20 and accumulates at an annual rate of 3.7%.[18] By age 80, the amount exceeds 30-50% of what it was in our twenties—which certainly necessitates the need to be an early adopter of good skin care practices and healthy lifestyle habits.

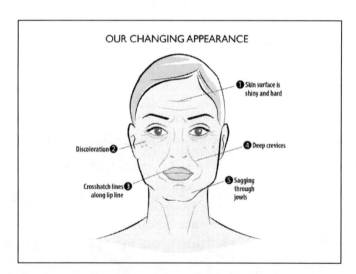

Unfortunately, there's more bad news. AGEs can bind to receptors on the surface of cells; these receptors for AGEs (RAGE) activate a series of biological reactions which indirectly and negatively impact skin. Cell proliferation, gene expression, and collagen and elastin synthesis can all be compromised. And as the acronym alludes to, albeit coincidentally, RAGE can induce oxidative stress and inflammation (inflammaging).

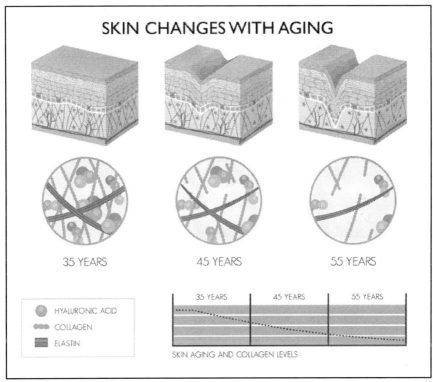

Inflammation is our body's natural protective reaction to an insult such as a wound, a virus, or bacteria. A complex symphony of cells and proteins participate in causing the classic signs of inflammation: redness, tenderness, heat, and swelling. When the offense is acute, the body usually does a good job in resolving the issue. The fire is extinguished. It's a different story when the offending agents—sugars, unhealthy fats, chemicals—are being constantly introduced. With these chronically present, inflammation smolders in the body.

Some Fats Fuel the Smoldering Fire
You've probably heard about the essential fatty acids, omega-6 fatty acids and omega-3 acids, and the generalization that omega-6 fats are "bad" and omega-3 fats are "good." I want to make it really simple—it's the imbalance between the two that gets us into the most trouble. Prior to the end of World War II and the introduction of the ubiquitous corn oil in

products, the ratio of omega-6/omega-3 was roughly two or three to one. This is a healthy ratio. For most people eating the SAD, this ratio has ballooned to twenty or thirty to one. In the next chapter, I'll delve into greater detail about which foods contain these essential fatty acids, but for now, I want to be clear that it's the overabundance of omega-6s in the SAD that are the bad guys. Omega-6s are the precursors to a type of protein called prostaglandins which stimulate pain receptors and promote inflammation.

Can the SAD Get Any More Sad?
Well, yes… it actually can and has. One consequence of modern farming has been the depletion of minerals from the soil. This is, of course, in addition to all the pesticides that have been sprayed onto food crops. Soil mineral loss causes foods to be lower in micronutrients that the body needs to catalyze enzymatic reactions. Loss of all types of minerals is common with conventional farming, but selenium, magnesium, and chromium are three of the big ones. And as we'll learn later on, these three minerals are critical for skin health and beauty.

Organic farming is less susceptible to mineral loss, and of course, no pesticides are applied during such farming, even though pesticide drift can occur. There has been some speculation that when chemical pesticides—which include herbicides and fungicides—are sprayed on farmland, the natural fungi in the soil are depleted. These are the same fungi that help plants absorb minerals and other nutrients from the soil. Furthermore, pesticides disrupt the symbiotic relationship between the bacteria and fungi in the soil—similar to the ecosystem of the gut microbiome.[19]

Whatever the reason that plant-based foods are losing minerals surely doesn't negate the fact that it is happening in many of the plant-based foods we rely upon for our own micronutrient intake. If increased agricultural efficiency (i.e., pesticide use) has led to nutrient deficiency, farmers markets and backyard gardens have new-found appeal for wellness-minded people.

THE RDAS: OPTIMAL VS. INSUFFICIENT VS. DEFICIENT

The Recommended Dietary Allowance (RDA) is the average amount of a specific vitamin or mineral that the FDA has deemed sufficient to meet the needs of healthy individuals in a particular age group and/or pregnancy status. Sadly, and due to the SAD, many Americans don't obtain the most basic nutrient intake—the Estimated Average Requirements (EARs), which are even less than the RDAs. And then there's the optimal nutrient level, which despite not being officially recognized by a regulatory agency, are supported by safety and efficacy studies. If you want glowing skin, you'll want an optimal intake of the nutrients that are right for you.

Even if you consume the RDAs, you may not be getting what you anticipate. Here's a few reasons why not:

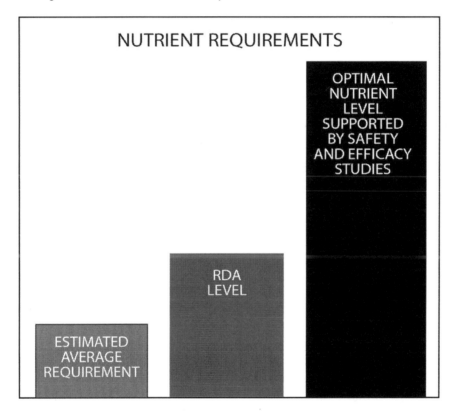

- Some vitamins in food get oxidized as they sit for days in the produce department or in your refrigerator, or after you've cooked them to a lovely army-green color.
- You may have a malabsorption issue which hampers the GI tract's ability to absorb and utilize a specific vitamin or mineral.
- You may have a genetic variant which predisposes you to a vitamin or mineral deficiency. (Refer to Chapter 5: Eating Right for Your Genes.)

- You may be taking a drug that interferes with the absorption or metabolism of a key nutrient. (See Chapter 11 for a list of drugs that interfere with nutrients.)

I've listed the RDAs for the vitamins and minerals most relevant to skin health in Appendix A. You'll also find the FDA's relevant information for insufficiency and deficiency, as well as excessive intake in Appendix B.

Don't Forget the Fiber

The SAD is dismally low in fiber, by virtue of its lack of fiber-rich vegetables, fruits, beans, whole grains, and nuts. And no, french fries and ketchup don't count! The average American adult eats a mere 15 grams of fiber per day. The recommendation is close to double that amount—25 grams for women and 38 grams for men. More is even better. Fiber-rich, plant-based foods supply the vitamins and minerals necessary for good health and good skin. In subsequent chapters, I'll explore the critical role that fiber plays in maintaining the health of the GI tract and "feeding" the good bacteria that inhabit the gut.

Avoid Fake Foods

In the effort to make our lives more convenient, food scientists have concocted "non-food" foods and food additives. These additives help extend shelf life (preservatives) and make foods more appetizing by improving taste, texture, and appearance (chemical flavorings, emulsifiers, dyes). Some even fill a practical need by reducing food waste or repurposing byproducts from other manufacturing processes. Laboratory-derived food substitutions, such as olestra for vegetable oils and aspartame for sugar, also earn the "fake" designation. While the original intent behind all these substitutions may have been good—getting salad dressings and ice cream to a uniform consistency with emulsifiers, say, or providing non-caloric sweeteners for people trying to lose weight or who have diabetes—we are now beginning to realize their deleterious effects on the gut microbiome.

Emulsifiers are blending agents for normally non-mixable ingredients, like oil and water, and they stabilize a food product, like a bottled salad dressing, so its ingredients will not separate. They also act as a preservative, so that store-bought ranch salad dressings last years, unlike freshly prepared vinaigrette. Natural emulsifiers, including egg yolks, honey, and mustard, are okay, but there are plenty of emulsifier ingredients in common processed foods, so you'll want to check the labels.

These additives can alter the composition of the gut microbiome, leading to systemic inflammation which in turn contributes to metabolic disease, obesity, inflammatory bowel disease (IBD), and various inflammatory-related skin conditions. As recently as 2015, researchers identified two specific emulsifiers—carboxymethylcellulose and polysorbate 80—as initiators of low-grade inflammation.[20] The use of synthetic emulsifiers has become ever present in processed foods, and researchers believe it is contributing to the increase in irritable bowel disease over the last 50 years.[21,22] Others have suggested that emulsifier alterations to the microbiome are powerful enough to promote tumor development, hence the concept of colitis-associated cancer.[23] Many foods marketed as "healthy" contain these unhealthy emulsifiers, particularly bars and energy drinks.

STAY AWAY FROM THESE COMMON EMULSIFIERS

- Carboxymethylcellulose
- Carrageenan
- Guar gum
- Locust bean gum
- Polyglycerols
- Polysorbate 80
- Soy lecithin
- Xanthan gum

Artificial sweeteners—with the possible exception of liquid stevia—are just about as fake as you can get even though they've been heavily promoted as "healthy lower calorie alternatives" to sugar. The calorie counting obsession has been steadily waning in the last decade thankfully, giving rise to the more sensible approach of tracking food quality. Unfortunately, diet sodas remain a mainstay of the SAD.

Aspartame (branded as NutraSweet® and Equal®) was not even developed as a sugar substitute in 1965, but rather as a drug to treat ulcers, and with a chemical name like aspartylphenylalanine-methyl-ester, it hardly says "healthy." Aspartame's accidental discovery, followed by a sordid FDA-approval history, still managed to propel its use into the American diet, with the buy-in from diet soda manufacturers being huge. Early disdain for aspartame came from its potential toxicity (retinal damage, birth defects, cancer) due to the methanol used to make it, which the human body converts into formaldehyde.

And then came along sucralose (branded as Splenda®) and acesulfame potassium (branded as Sweet One®) as "healthier alternatives" to aspartame. Incidentally, consumer demand appears to have sparked aspartame's return because diet soda drinkers did not like the aftertaste of sucralose. The current disdain for artificial sweeteners in general comes from the disruption (dysbiosis) they cause to the gut microbiota; researchers have observed this effect with aspartame, sucralose, and saccharin (Sweet'N Low®).[24] People who consume diet drinks and diet foods have an increased risk of insulin resistance, type 2 diabetes, and inflammatory-related skin conditions, such as acne and rosacea.

> You would do well to remember that people with really good skin eat real foods. So, don't eat it if:
>
> - You can't pronounce it.
> - You can't identify the original plant or animal source.
> - It was made in a lab.
> - It has an unnatural color.
> - It sounds really scary.

FOOD SENSITIVITIES

One Person's Food is Another's "Poison"

OK, you avoid sugar as much as possible, and you are working to get more healthy fats into your diet, but you're still not happy with your skin. You have occasional breakouts, excessive dryness, or splotchy red skin. You suspect that it might be something you're eating (because, say, it happens every time you eat strawberries). Foods we once enjoyed as children now make us "react" in some way and our skin reflects it. Have we changed? Or is it that the foods we eat today have changed? It's a little of both. (Think: *pesticides* on those strawberries.) The science of skin health now takes into account food sensitivities—food allergies, food reactions, and food intolerances.

The prevalence of food sensitivities has been on the rise for quite some time. Twenty-five to 33% of people report that they react in some way to eating a particular food.[25] These reactions result from a combination of factors—digestive imbalances, genetics, and environment—all of which are unique to each individual. As for the foods themselves, food additives (i.e., MSG, sulfites, food dyes), food processing, pesticide application, and genetic modification contribute to reactions in susceptible people. When ingested, the immune system mistakes an otherwise harmless substance for a serious threat and initiates a reaction against it.

I want to clarify the difference between **true food allergies, delayed response reactions,** and **food intolerances** because these terms are frequently used interchangeably but not accurately.

A true food allergy occurs shortly after ingesting a particular food (rapid onset). In the worst case, this may elicit a severe and potentially life-threatening reaction (anaphylaxis). Food allergies are mediated by the immune system's IgE antibodies. Individuals can experience a wide range of symptoms with varying degrees of severity, including itching or tingling in the mouth; swelling of the face, lips, gums, tongue, or throat; difficulty breathing; itchy skin with or without hives or eczema; abdominal pain, nausea, vomiting, or diarrhea; and light-headedness, dizziness, or fainting. An allergist or immunologist should formally diagnose, treat, and manage patients with true food allergies due to the anaphylactic potential and risk of death. Food allergies are more common in children; some may outgrow them by adulthood, but in general, the body recognizes (and reacts to) the allergens throughout life.

Delayed response food reactions are significantly less severe, but nonetheless cause unpleasant symptoms. They are mediated by IgG (most common), IgA, and IgM antibodies of the immune system. These reactions typically occur further away from the time of ingestion (up to a few days), are dose dependent and temporary, and symptoms are often limited to GI symptoms. Most people experience bloating, flatulence, constipation, and/or diarrhea. That being said, some people can experience skin rashes, acne, arthritis, widespread body pain, headaches, fatigue, mood swings, irritability, and brain fog. Food reactions occur at any age and often change throughout one's life. The influence of how our food is grown and processed may play a key role in whether or not we're able to enjoy our favorite foods.

Food intolerances are related to enzyme insufficiencies which inhibit or prevent the breakdown of a certain element within a food (i.e., lactose, fructose). In turn, these elements cannot be absorbed properly into the body. This results in symptoms that frequently mimic irritable bowel syndrome (IBS), such as constipation, diarrhea, abdominal spasms, flatulence, and nausea. Lactose intolerance is probably the most common and well-known intolerance—caused by an insufficiency of the enzyme lactase which helps break down the sugar (lactose) in milk and other dairy products. However, both lactose intolerance and milk protein allergy can produce multiple skin symptoms.

Hereditary fructose intolerance is relatively rare, yet many people are just not that tolerant of fructose, particularly because it has become a big part of the American diet (i.e., high fructose corn syrup, fruit juices). Fructose intolerance is often misdiagnosed as IBS.

LACTOSE INTOLERANCE VS. MILK PROTEIN ALLERGY

INTOLERANCE (more common)	**ALLERGY** (less common)
Pain or abdominal cramps	Commonly diagnosed in infancy
Stomach gurgling or rumbling sounds	Eczema, rash, hives
Gas/flatulence	Severe diarrhea
Diarrhea or loose stools	Frequent ear infections
Vomiting	Difficult breathing
Diaper rash in babies	Wheezing, sneezing
	Swelling of the lips, gums, mouth, tongue, throat, face

Take Stock of Your Food Allergies

Functional medicine doctors, nutritionists or dietitians are typically the professionals that patients turn to when they suspect food sensitivities or intolerances, although a DIY approach can be effective. The gold standard for diagnosing food allergies is the elimination diet. You avoid the most common food-related triggers known to cause sensitivities for a three to four-week period. You then gradually add them back into the diet, one at a time, over a period of several days—and monitor how you react.

If you are disciplined, this can be an excellent self-care tool. Due to the elusive nature of identifying the specific cause of a sensitivity, a new food should be added back once every three days. Your healthcare practitioner may also want to order professional food sensitivity blood tests, which may check for elevations in IgE and/or IgG. As most of these tests are not insurance reimbursable, you'll want to clearly understand the costs and benefits in conversation with your clinician.

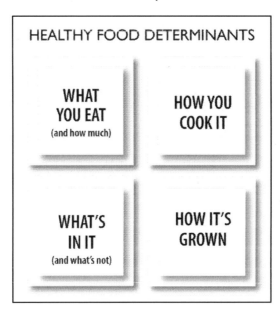

Increasingly, companies such as Everlywell (everlywell.com) are marketing large IgG panels (for ~90 to 200 foods) directly to consumers. The difficult comes in interpreting the results. Adam Silberman, ND, a functional medicine practitioner in San Diego notes, "It can be challenging for patients to integrate the results of IgG testing into their lives. Especially if a number of foods come up. They can get stuck thinking 'I can't eat anything!' Often, when many foods come back positive on an IgG test, it can be a sign of intestinal permeability. The non-fully digested food products make their way into the bloodstream and aggravate the immune system. This may not necessarily reflect a true sensitivity to the food itself. Working with a practitioner can be very helpful in implementing the results of the testing, understanding what is a true food sensitivity versus what could be a sign of intestinal permeability. We work with patients to decide how long to avoid the foods found to be problematic on a panel, and how to reintroduce them." Dr. Silberman also finds food sensitivity testing a very effective tool in addressing skin conditions from acne to eczema. "I also recommend food sensitivity testing prior to aesthetic

> **COMMON TRIGGERS OF FOOD ALLERGIES & SENSITIVITIES**
>
> - Grains, especially wheat (gluten)
> - Dairy products (lactose)
> - Eggs, typically egg whites
> - Peanuts
> - Soy
> - Tree nuts
> - Shellfish
> - Nightshades (tomatoes, potatoes, eggplant, hot/sweet peppers)
> - Corn
> - Sugar (fructose)
> - Chemicals and additives used in processed foods

procedures like skin resurfacing, PRP, or surgery, as outcomes are better and recovery time is shorter if patients can avoid the offending foods."

With all the buzz around gluten and a bevy of gluten-free foods and restaurants catering to the gluten-free lifestyle, non-celiac gluten sensitivity (NCGS) has emerged as a real condition, separate from celiac disease. Celiac disease affects approximately 1% of Americans, and NCGS affects up to 6%.[26] Despite these relatively low percentages, a Gallup poll showed that twenty percent of Americans actively include gluten-free foods in their diets.[27] To confuse things a bit further, one study suggested that some people with self-reported NCGS actually had a fructan (fructooligosaccharides) sensitivity.[28]

Fructans are found in several non-gluten-containing foods such as agave, artichokes, asparagus, garlic, leeks, jicama, onions, and yacón, as well as the gluten-containing foods barley and wheat. This points to the challenging nature of getting to the bottom of one's symptoms and why an elimination diet may help. We'll discuss more about how gluten—in sensitive individuals—can worsen leaky gut syndrome, alter the microbiome, and lead to inflammation in the body.

Great Skin Depends on Great Nutrition

Now that we've identified the bad actors that play a role in skin health, let's talk *skin* and what happens as we advance chronologically (which, by the way, begins the day we're born).

Aging is a complex process which involves the loss and compromise of various cellular functions. Skin cells lose their ability to divide and make new skin cells. The mitochondria (energy powerhouses) within the skin cells diminish with age. They also become dysfunctional and lose their ability to generate energy. The ability of skin cells to do their internal housekeeping (autophagy) is affected. Blood flow which delivers vital nutrients and oxygen to keep skin cells nourished and hydrated is compromised. These same processes also occur in most cells of the human body as we age, yet lifestyle can accelerate or decelerate the rate of change. Most people never see an aging liver or kidney, but they do see aging skin every time they look into a mirror.

Getting Inside Your Skin

The skin is one of the fastest growing organs in the body. It generates new cells from the basal layer of the epidermis, the section of the skin that lies just above the dermis. The dermis contains blood vessels, nerves, sweat glands, hair follicles, all held together by an extracellular matrix (ECM) that is rich in collagen and elastin.

The rate at which the skin turns over—when new cells from the basal layer reach the outermost layer of your body—varies among individuals. The skin regenerates continuously throughout your life. It is estimated that, in humans, the epidermis turns over every 40–56 days, and for comparison, in mice, it's 8–10 days.[29] That may keep the mice looking forever youthful, but sadly for them, they don't get to live as long as we do. If one of the hallmarks of aging is slow skin turnover, accompanied by an accumulation of dull, lifeless, horny-looking skin cells on the surface of the skin, how do we supercharge the skin's innate ability to regenerate itself and transform—slow, halt, or reverse—aging skin into youthful, vibrant, soft as-a-baby skin?

Healthy skin cell turnover depends on robust circulation of the nutrient-rich blood flowing to skin tissues—those same nutrients that come from your diet. This is why feeding your skin from within is so critical if you want young, glowing skin. In Chapter 2: Choose This Not That–Making the Most of Your Diet, I'll review the eating habits that are best for skin health, including the types of macronutrients and micronutrients science has shown to be most beneficial for most people. Keep in mind that even if a food is deemed "good for the skin," not every person's skin reacts to it positively.

Chapter 2

CHOOSE THIS NOT THAT – MAKING THE MOST OF YOUR DIET

Now that you've examined your diet for the bad actors, considered possible food reactions, and have a general understanding of how nutrition affects the skin, it's time to take action. I've written *Feed Your Skin Right* to coincide with the nutritional needs (what/how should I eat?) of *all* people, *some* people, and ultimately *you*! To this end, I'll provide some guidance for several nutrition-related chronic skin conditions such as acne, psoriasis, and eczema. Later, in Chapters 4 and 5, I'll discuss how an individual's gut microbiome and genes can influence his or her personalized nutritional needs. But let's start with the basics: what happens when you put food in your mouth.

Digestion. Absorption. Metabolism.
The process of eating well begins in your head. This is known as the "cephalic" phase of digestion. Basically, it is the time before we eat in which we ideally slow down, relax, smell our food, and anticipate the many tastes to come. This activity helps to initiate the digestive process and jump-starts the enzymes, nerves, and hormones that orchestrate the highly coordinated process of getting nutrients into your body.

If you want to feed your skin right, you'll need to ensure that what you put into your mouth actually reaches your skin. In other words, you can't put the cart (great nutrient-rich foods) before the horses (digestion, absorption, and metabolism) and expect healthy skin. Enzymes are key to how well the body functions overall and are necessary components to chemical reactions in every cell. With respect to eating food, digestive enzymes break down carbohydrates, fats, and proteins into smaller units which the body can absorb as fuel. They're produced primarily by the pancreas, but also the liver, gallbladder, stomach, small intestine, and colon. The amylase, lipase, and protease enzymes are native to the human body. Cellulase is an enzyme that is not produced by the body, rather, some nutritional supplements add it to their mixture.

- Amylase breaks down plant-based carbohydrates and starches
- Lipase breaks down animal and plant-based fats
- Protease breaks down animal and plant-based proteins
- Cellulase breaks down plant fiber

Equally important are the metabolic enzymes which control the speed of the cells' chemical reactions. Without them, food digestion would be way too slow to be efficient.

Since great skin begins with your first bite of food, it's important to chew well. As you chew, glands in the mouth and esophagus release saliva which contains enzymes necessary for digestion. Two major salivary enzymes—salivary amylase (breaks down starches) and lingual lipase (breaks down fats) jumpstart the digestive process, so the more chewing the better. By extension, strong teeth and good oral health are influential in maintaining good skin.

Once food reaches the stomach, it's met with an even stronger digestive aid—gastric juice, which includes hydrochloric acid, pepsin, and intrinsic factor. Hydrochloric acid (HCl) is perhaps most well-known for creating the stomach's acidic environment. Combined with mechanical digestive processes, gastric juice helps foster optimized nutrient absorption by the time food reaches the small intestine. HCl has another important job of killing pathogenic bacteria and viruses that have hitched a ride with your food or in contaminated water. The enzyme pepsin helps digest the proteins found in meat, dairy, eggs, nuts, and seeds into amino acids. Intrinsic factor binds to vitamin B12 in the stomach before traveling to the small intestine where the B12 is absorbed.

As some people get older, the amount of HCl produced by the stomach decreases, and one of two conditions can develop. A lack of HCl—called *achlorhydria*—and reduced HCl—called *hypochlorhydria*—occur in people less than 60 years at rates of 2.3% and 2% respectively, but increase to 5% in the over-sixty age group.[30] Both achlorhydria and hypochlorhydria are more common in patients with gastrointestinal diseases and/or autoimmune diseases. These two conditions compromise food digestion and absorption, while increasing susceptibility to gut-based infections (i.e., food poisoning).

Enzyme production can also taper off with age. The telltale symptoms of decreased enzyme secretion include bloating, gas, indigestion, heartburn, and irregularity, and although these can be occasional and unrelated to digestive enzymes, nearly one of every three Americans experience these symptoms on a daily basis. For example: If you have a lactase deficiency, which impairs lactose (sugar in milk) breakdown, you'll experience lactose intolerance (bloating and gas) when you consume milk and other dairy products. Furthermore, naturally-occurring enzymes in plant-based foods are destroyed in processed foods and grains—another great reason for minimizing processed foods!

Daily enzyme supplementation is a simple, safe, and effective way to reduce your digestive distress and improve regularity. I recommend Enzymedica® products for this purpose (enzymedica.com), with my favorite being DigestGold™. Supplementing with enzymes does not interfere with your body's own natural production of enzymes. We all have an "enzyme potential" which is the amount our body will create in our lifetime. Supplementing can substantially increase the longevity of what you naturally make. It does this by storing what your body produces so the enzymes can be used in other chemical functions.

Alternatively, you can take digestive bitters (Angostura® is most well-known) before a meal; these induce the flow of saliva, digestive enzymes, and stomach acid, thereby priming the GI tract to break down food. With consistent use, you'll feel more energetic, less uncomfortable, and you'll maximize the skin benefits of the foods you eat.

BITTERS GET THINGS FLOWING
Place 20 drops in a ¼ cup of slightly warmed water. Sip slowly 5 minutes before eating a meal.

WHAT SHOULD MOST OF US EAT?
Foods and beverages contain macronutrients—the "big" nutrients—like carbohydrates, protein, and fats, which the body breaks down into glucose (sugar), amino acids, and fatty acids. These are the nutrients that provide the energy (calories), that the body needs to function—sort of like the gas

you put in your car. If your vehicle manufacturer recommends premium unleaded gas, this is the blend to make the engine run smooth and efficiently. So, you opt to spend a little extra for premium, and avoid the temptation to put in a lower grade of fuel. It's the same with your body; give it the best fuel you can afford. (Of course, this analogy will be useless when we all drive electric cars—and it bolsters my assertion that the truth as we know it today is likely to be different tomorrow.) While there will always be some disagreement as to what are the "best" foods, there are a set of principles that apply to all of us.

Eat Lower on the Food Chain

A more plant-based diet with less meat consumption typifies the idea behind "eating lower on the food chain." Of course, this means different things to different people—from veganism, to vegetarianism, to pescatarianism, to "Fish-day Friday," and "Meatless Mondays." Each of these eating styles offers some benefits to both personal health and to the health of our environment. The natural resources needed to grow fruits and vegetables is significantly lower than that of raising conventional livestock, and the body's protein requirements can be adequately supplied by eating mostly plant-based foods, provided that pure vegetarians and vegans complement their proteins. If you're committed to eating at the bottom of the food chain, keep in mind that most plant proteins are less digestible than animal proteins and thus, less easily absorbed in the body.

In order to build a complete protein, the body needs all the essential amino acids that come from the diet. For vegetarians and vegans, combining grains and legumes, and adding nuts and seeds rich in the amino acids tryptophan, methionine, and cysteine, will provide ample building blocks for the body. Some nutrients such as protein, iron, calcium, zinc, vitamin B12 and vitamin D can be harder to obtain from a vegetarian or vegan diet and may require supplementation for optimal health. If you are occasionally consuming eggs, dairy, fish, seafood, or animal protein, your protein requirements will be satisfied.

How Much Protein Do I Need?

You can already anticipate the answer: *It depends*. It depends upon your age, your activity level, and your goals. While we most commonly think of protein being the food source for the looking-good muscles like the abs, biceps, and quads, it is also necessary to maintain the facial muscles as well as the muscles of the neck. It's essential for skin, healthy hair and nails. Amino acids, the byproducts of protein metabolism, are critical not just for muscle, but also for the synthesis of hormones and neurotransmitters.

One of the hallmarks of aging is the gradual loss of muscle mass with age. After the age of 30, the average person loses approximately 3–8% per decade. This rate of decline accelerates for those 60 years old or more.[31]

The basic Recommended Dietary Allowance (RDA) for protein is set at 0.8 grams of protein per kilogram of body weight. A kilogram is 2.2 pounds, so a 144 lb. person would weigh 70 kilograms, and have a protein recommendation of 56 grams per day. However, this level of protein is inadequate for athletes. The Academy of Nutrition and Dietetics, Dietitians of Canada and the American College of Sports Medicine recommend, depending upon training, that athletes take in 1.2 to 2.0 grams of protein per kilogram of body weight per day, spaced throughout the day.

GOOD SOURCES OF PLANT-BASED PROTEIN

BEANS	PEAS	SEEDS	OTHER
Lentils	Split peas	Hemp	Quinoa
Black beans	Green peas	Pumpkin	Wild rice
Lima beans	Chickpeas	Sacha Inchi	Buckwheat
Kidney Beans		Chia	
Navy beans		Sunflower	
Pinto beans			

Get Closer to the Source

Growing food in your backyard or in a community garden has its benefits—relaxation, stress management, light exercise, and of course, better tasting and more nutritious fruits and vegetables. And one sure thing: You know *where* your food came from and *when* it came to your table, unlike the supermarket guessing game. Some of my early beliefs about food reflect how detached I really was from the source of my daily meals. It wasn't until the COVID-19 pandemic that I realized time spent at home in lockdown could nurture a budding green thumb.

I was raised in the blue-collar suburbs of Long Island, New York, where my major understanding of food growing up was that meat came on Styrofoam covered by cellophane. Vegetables were either frozen, or from a can. As the oldest of three boys, I was tasked with heating up the TV dinners for us when my parents had to work late. Needless to say, growing up I never really got close to the source of where food comes from. I once tried growing a garden when I was young, but to my chagrin, the ducks in our backyard were better harvesters than I was.

It wasn't until the pandemic that I finally got into the joys of gardening. Instead of flying 150,000 miles a year, I was grounded. My passion was initially fueled by the gift of an AeroGarden® (aerogarden.com), a self-contained growing platform in which you insert seeded pods into a device that waters and lights the plants automatically. The best thing is that the entire device took up less than 2 square feet and produced a plethora of herbs and veggies in a matter of weeks. Fired up from my AeroGarden® success, I went to ground—making raised beds, composting, fertilizing, weeding, and pruning. Today, I take it as a higher compliment that my tomatoes are "delicious" than that my talk at a conference was "wonderful." My only regret is that I didn't instill this same love into the DNA of my children when they were growing up. (They still turned out well.)

Every so often, I come across these "Duh" articles that ask, Should Children be Taught to Grow Food in School?[32] Duh, because this is a no-brainer; the answer is an absolute "yes." When children actively participate in growing their own organic food, they develop an appreciation for organically grown produce as well as for the people who grow food, and are more likely to eat (and enjoy) their vegetables. They're also more likely to adopt healthier eating habits because of the positive nutrition beliefs and attitudes gained or reinforced through their hands-on gardening experience.

Eat Clean

Prior to the discovery and use of chemical pesticides, of which herbicides like glyphosate are a sub-type, foods were organic and wholesome. People ate without worry. Then mass spraying of pesticides came along, and people *still* ate without worry—because they were told that pesticides helped grow more food and made food more readily available to more people at a lower cost. With the ubiquitous use of pesticides in conventional farming operations today, the notion of "lower cost" is arguably quite different today.

The "health cost" has surreptitiously affected Americans even when they believe they're eating organic. Arial spraying of pesticides can lead to pesticide drift that reaches far beyond the original farm. Crops on neighboring organic farms can be affected depending upon which way the wind blows. A "certified organic" farm can still produce foods with low levels of contamination, and although consumers are unlikely to know, it doesn't mean you should give up on organics either. Eat organic whenever possible and make purchases from reputable vendors, farmers markets, or grow your own. Your microbiome and the gut-brain-skin axis will thank you for it. To help you make better produce choices, the Environmental Working Group offers their "Dirty 12" and "Clean 15."[33]

THE DIRTY DOZEN	THE CLEAN FIFTEEN
1. Strawberries	1. Avocados
2. Spinach	2. Sweet corn
3. Kale, collard & mustard greens	3. Pineapple
	4. Onions
4. Nectarines	5. Papaya
5. Apples	6. Sweet peas (frozen)
6. Grapes	7. Eggplant
7. Cherries	8. Asparagus
8. Peaches	9. Broccoli
9. Pears	10. Cabbage
10. Bell & hot peppers	11. Kiwi
11. Celery	12. Cauliflower
12. Tomatoes	13. Mushrooms
	14. Honeydew melon
	15. Cantaloupe

Go Low, Not High

High glycemic foods such as sodas, fruit juice beverages, candy, cakes, pastries, and other confections are notoriously high in simple sugars and white flour which the body rapidly breaks down into glucose. The glycemic index is a ranking of common foods by how quickly they raise blood sugar levels; the scale applies to foods that contain carbohydrates, not pure protein or fat sources. All foods are compared to pure glucose, which has a score of 100. Your dietary goal should be to primarily consume foods that are ranked either low or medium on the glycemic index. This means choosing whole foods and eliminating the processed foods, fast foods, and white foods (white sugar, white flour, white bread, white rice, white pasta, white potatoes, etc.).

In addition to the glycemic index, there is also a glycemic load (GL) ranking which takes into consideration average portion size, which the glycemic index does not. The values for both rankings are shown below.

GLYCEMIC INDEX	GLYCEMIC LOAD
Low GI: 55 or less	Low GL: 10 or less
Medium GI: 56-69	Medium GL: 11-19
High GI: 70 or higher	High GL: 20 or higher

With the advent of continuous glucose monitoring (a recording patch that adheres to your arm and detects blood glucose), it is possible to record personalized data right on your smart phone. There are a number of companies that have created excellent systems including Levels (levels-health.com), January AI (january.ai), and Nutrisense (nutrisense.io). After using one of these systems for four weeks, you'll wind up with a solid program to manage your blood sugar through intelligent food choices. For those who must frequently make food choices on the go, most nutritionists suggest examining the label and choosing products with 6 grams or less of sugar.

The Health Consequences of Too Much Sugar

Aside from being a prime target for glycation, excess glucose can be stored as fat. Over time, excess fat storage leads to obesity and other health complications. Among these complications, insulin resistance (abnormal glucose metabolism, often leading to pre-diabetes and type 2 diabetes) is particularly concerning. Insulin resistance has been implicated as a contributor to skin inflammation and acne vulgaris.[34] Obesity is a risk factor for psoriasis, and additional weight gain may cause flare-ups in people who already have psoriasis.[35]

When all is said and done, the body converts all carbohydrates, even the low glycemic carbs, into glucose, albeit at a much slower than it does for high glycemic foods. Glucose will signal your pancreas to pump out higher insulin levels. Too much insulin causes insulin resistance—which means the body stops adequately responding to insulin and more and more insulin gets produced in the body's attempt to get rid of sugar from the bloodstream. As a result, you pack more fat and blood sugar goes up. Naturally, with the rising incidence of obesity, insulin resistance is also on the rise. So, in general, go easy on all carbs. If you can't give up your mid-morning latte and scone cold turkey, cut your consumption in half (and in half again) and choose low glycemic alternatives instead. By cutting back, the amount of fuel for inflammation and glycation will be greatly reduced. If the thought of developing type 2 diabetes doesn't scare you, maybe the premature and excessive wrinkle formation will.

Go for the Essential Fats

Eating good quality essential fats goes hand-in-hand with reducing high glycemic carbs while focusing on non-starchy, nutrient-dense vegetables instead. The essential fats, or essential fatty acids (EFAs), are called "essential" because the body can't make them, but it certainly does need them, so they must be supplied by the diet. EFAs are foundational to the cell membrane—and of every cell membrane in the body, especially the skin cells. If your skin is dry and flaky, it's probably deficient in EFAs.

Because the body can't manufacture EFAs, we must obtain them from food. The best sources are plant-based healthy fats such as extra virgin olive oil and avocado oil as well as fatty fish such as wild-caught salmon, mackerel, sardines, and anchovies. Of all the diet trends today, the Mediterranean eating style is the most advantageous for a healthy microbiome and overall skin health. This can be attributed to the high content of omega-3 fatty acids and some of the beneficial omega-6 fatty acids within the foods favored by this diet. Both types of fats play an important role in skin function and skin appearance.[36]

Omega-3s are a type of polyunsaturated fat that you should think of as your "best friend" because they help reduce inflammation throughout the body and benefit the gut-brain-skin axis. Specifically, in the skin, omega-3s help control oil production and nourish the skin cell membranes. This serves to prevent acne in acne-prone individuals, provide a strong barrier to keep toxins out, and slow skin aging by hydrating the skin and staving off wrinkles. The most important omega-3s are eicosapentaenoic acid (EPA) and docosahexaenoic acid (DHA)—found in fish—and alphalinolenic acid (ALA)—found in nuts and seeds. One of the easiest ways to get additional omega-3s is to sprinkle foods with ground flax seeds. They impart a wonderful, nutty flavor to foods and are easy to store in your refrigerator.

Omega-3s have a set of cousins—the omega-6s, also a group of polyunsaturated fats which play a role in maintaining the skin's barrier. But, unlike the "friendly" omega-3s, their omega-6 cousins are not so friendly and, having been corrupted by manufacturing processes, are proinflammatory. Processed omega-6s are found in corn oil, canola oil, safflower oil, soybean oil, and sunflower oil. These oils are prevalent in the American diet and although the body needs some omega-6s, they should be minimized and only from natural, unmodified sources.

It has been suggested that a ketogenic or paleo diet—by virtue of being low-carb and low-sugar—improves skin appearance or reduces acne in some people. This may instead be due to people losing weight and lowering insulin resistance. However, others contend that the high-protein, high-fat eating style lacks enough fiber for the gut bacteria to thrive. And with limited vitamins from vegetables and fruits, deficiencies may develop. These same vitamins are mediators of good skin health. Ketogenic or paleo diets may be valuable in the short-term to achieve a healthy body weight and reduce the risk of diabetes, but in the long-term, a different eating style may be more advantageous to great looking skin.

The Pegan Diet proposed by Mark Hyman, MD in 2014 is more of a paleo-vegan hybrid that takes advantage of the best features from each. Dr. Hyman recommends eating 75% plant and fiber-based produce and 25% grass-fed, pasture- and sustainably-raised meat. The key to "healthy beef" is that when cows graze naturally on grass in the fields, they eat natural omega-3s, so that their meat contains more omega-3s than omega-6s. Farm-raised salmon can suffer a similar fate, so be certain to choose the wild-caught version.

Fill Your Plate with Color

One of the leading nutritionists in the country, Deanna Minich, PhD, has created a wellness lifestyle program (deannaminich.com) by which she encourages people to "Eat in Color." She's a Functional Medicine Practitioner whose expertise in nutritional biochemistry reminds me to fill my plate with the colors of the rainbow at every major meal. No more monochrome meals staring back at you! Colorful vegetables and fruits contain a plethora of phytonutrients.

Carotenoid pigments like beta-carotene (a precursor of vitamin A), lycopene, lutein, and vitamin A itself play a role in preventing skin damage caused by UV exposure and pollution. As antioxidants, these substances help neutralize inflammation when the skin is over-exposed to sunlight. They also promote skin cell turnover in which dead skin cells are sloughed off and new skin cells appear. Vitamin C helps fortify the skin's collagen and elastin to maintain a youthful appearance. Glutathione helps skin cells fight free radical damage caused by life's stressors. Vitamin A assists in wound healing by regulating the growth of skin cells and enhances collagen production.[37]

TOP CONTENDERS FOR NUTRIENT-SKIN BENEFITS

- Dark leafy greens – spinach, kale, chard, collard greens
- Carrots, winter squash, mango, watermelon
- Asparagus
- Avocados
- Cooked tomatoes
- Citrus fruits – oranges, grapefruit, lemons, limes
- Berries

Consider the Dairy Dilemma

I recognize that some folks may be averse to dairy consumption, but milk "can do a body good" for most people. It's a good source of protein and is packed with valuable nutrients such as calcium, riboflavin, vitamins A, D, B1, and B12, magnesium, potassium, phosphorus, selenium, and zinc. A good option for milk drinkers is to choose milk that comes from grass-fed or pasture-raised cows; their milk contains higher quantities of omega-3 fatty acids and other beneficial antioxidants than conventionally-raised dairy cows.

Dairy products are prime suspects in the development of skin inflammation and acne, but with the final word still pending, there's an increasing belief that skim milk may be the real culprit. Research finds that people who drink either skim or low-fat have a higher incidence of acne,[38] suggesting this is related to two milk proteins—whey and casein—that are added back to improve the texture (i.e., make it less watery). Whey affects insulin secretion, thereby hindering adequate blood glucose control and fueling inflammation. Casein may trigger an immune response in susceptible individuals which increases inflammation.

Since whole milk contains whey and casein, but a lesser amount, eliminate milk and ice cream if you experience acne. If you're a skim milk drinker and you don't want to go full-fat, try a plant-based milk alternative. Athletes and other people who frequently drink whey protein shakes and/or consume protein bars are more prone to acne. Protein bars can be high in sugar, too, so check the labels. Plain, unsweetened yogurt and cheese do not appear to be problematic, which might be due to fermentation and aging processes. Avoiding dairy for 2-3 weeks as part of a modified elimination diet will provide clues on just how your body responds.

SHINING LIGHT ON DARK CHOCOLATE

You've probably heard that dark chocolate (70% or more cacao) is good for you. Cacao is rich in a type of antioxidant known as epicatechin. In the scientific literature, the bioactive ingredient is the negatively charged form, or -epicatechin. -Epicatechin has a positive effect on maintaining the integrity of the endothelium, most notably the lining of vessels in the heart. It exerts positive effects in the mitochondria and other cells through providing more nitric oxide.[39]

Most commercial chocolate bars; however, are loaded with excess sugar and unhealthy fats. As a lifelong chocolate connoisseur, I've landed on one produced by Hu: Get Back to Human® (hukitchen.com). Their bars contain no emulsifiers, no soy lecithin, no dairy, and no refined sugar. They use organic unrefined coconut sugar (still a sugar, but not as processed). I have one or two small squares of the Salty Dark Chocolate every day around 3 pm as a wonderful pick me up.

Going one step further, many companies are evaluating the use of chocolate as a carrier to deliver bioactive ingredients.[40] One such company that's pioneered a line of bite sized chocolates is FX Chocolate (fxchocolate.com). Their product line includes a variety of bioactives such as melatonin, reishi mushroom extracts, ashwagandha, vitamin D_3, and vitamin K2.

Both products are not inexpensive. However, when it comes to a treat, I'd rather ingest small amounts of a higher quality product than large amounts of an inferior one.

TIME YOUR EATING

Lately, there's been increased awareness of interest in various forms of time-restricted feeding (TRF) for both weight loss, as well as general health benefits. With TRF you limit the daily period of food intake to 8-10 hours or less most days of the week. You are "fasting" the other 14-16 hours. This can help you cut down on calories. Another type of TRF, Intermittent fasting (IMF) cuts calories down by 60% or more 2-5 days a week. So, a person who would normally eat a 2,000 calorie diet would only consume 500 calories for the days of the fast. For those who are interested in weight loss, both methods yield about the same results.[41]

Fasting, in general, has been utilized by health-conscious individuals for its purported health benefits, especially weight control, weight loss, and detoxification. It is an integral part of several religious traditions and cultural or ethnic rituals and ceremonies. You could even say that the practice of fasting—albeit unintended—dates back tens of thousands of years to a time when food was scarce. The "3 square meals a day" is a historically new concept, which may, in part, contribute to the current crisis related to over-feeding—obesity, cardiovascular disease, and type 2 diabetes.

One of the most advantageous, somewhat newly discovered health benefits is that fasting (and general calorie restriction) helps improve insulin sensitivity and decreases inflammation. Of course, the non-fasting periods should not be rife with refined sugars, starches, and processed foods which are also abundant in chemicals and artificial additives, nor should they be filled with extra calories to make up for what was not consumed during the fasting period. Reduced insulin sensitivity and increased inflammation caused by an unhealthy diet can play a role in poor physical and mental health, chronic disease, and some inflammatory-related skin conditions. Once again, we look to the gut-brain-skin axis because as we know, a happy gut and happy brain make for happy and beautiful skin.

One of the key physiological effects induced by fasting is known as *autophagy*. Autophagy is a process of cellular housekeeping which cleans up the "waste products" in the body's cells, such as damaged mitochondria, and recycles them into new functional components for the cells. You can think of autophagy as the housekeeping staff at your hotel coming in and cleaning up after your previous day's mess. Their efficiency allows you to return to a freshly cleaned and orderly room. The optimal time for autophagy is during sleep, when the body naturally detoxifies and repairs itself. Hetal Patel, MD, a fellowship-trained integrative physician in San Diego, always reminds his patients that there should be a hyphen between break and fast; break-fast.

Sleep is a natural state of fasting. In other words, you don't normally eat while you're sleeping, and your body's glucose stores diminish throughout the night. If you do happen to sleepwalk to the refrigerator or you consciously go for that midnight snack, then you break your natural fast. So, instead of being in a detoxification-repair state, your body goes into a digestive state. Whether you ate a pint of ice cream or a piece of fruit, the body's glucose stores are replenished to some degree (depending on how much you ate and how easily it was converted to glucose).

> ### DON'T SKIMP ON SLEEP
> The body requires sleep for a variety of reasons, not just autophagy, but the key, however, is *restorative* sleep. Most adults need 7 or more hours of quality sleep every night for optimal functioning. If you're not getting this currently, prioritize your sleep as part of your skincare regimen.[42]

Time-restricted feeding helps encourage autophagy, while simultaneously promoting another potentially useful metabolic process in the body—ketosis. In a nutshell, ketosis occurs when the body's cells utilize dietary fat and stored fat calories (body fat) for fuel instead of glucose. The various ketogenic ("keto") diets are based on the premise of obtaining more of one's daily calories from protein and fat sources, rather than carbohydrates, especially the carbs that are easily converted to glucose (bread, baked goods, candy, soda, rice). When fat is the primary fuel source, ketones are produced, which happen to be a favored fuel for the brain. During a fast—at any time of the day or night—ketosis begins when the glucose stores are depleted. For most people, ketosis kicks in after about 12 hours of fasting. This is the reason that TRF protocols require 12, 14, 16, or 18 hours of fasting.

My preferred TRF-keto diet is KetoFLEX 12/3, the plan espoused by Dale E. Bredesen, MD.[43] Dr. Bredesen is an expert in the field of neurodegeneration and the prevention/reversal of Alzheimer's disease through nutrition and eating habits. Maintaining mitochondrial health is essential to cognitive (brain) health, and that's where autophagy, reduced inflammation, and improved insulin sensitivity come in. The KetoFLEX 12/3 plan is a medically sound strategy for attaining mild ketosis daily.

Here's how the fasting component works:
- Fast for a minimum of **12** hours from the time you take your last dinner bite to your first breakfast bite.
- Fast for **3** to 4 hours before going to bed. Permitted beverages during this time include plain water, decaffeinated black coffee, or green tea.
- Break the fast by drinking a glass of room temperature water with some fresh-squeezed lemon juice or a cup of herbal tea (ginger, lemongrass, dandelion, or milk thistle).

The KetoFLEX 12/3 plan is easy for most people to follow and over time, many find themselves increasing the fasting time beyond 12 hours. This can be achieved by reducing the "3 square meals a day" to just 2 meals. Depending on preference, this might mean skipping breakfast or dinner, or having an earlier and lighter dinner.

The neurocognitive benefits of the KetoFLEX 12/3 plan will continue to be borne out as time passes, but what does intermittent fasting have to do with beautiful, younger-looking skin? Quite a lot, actually, and I think by this point, you probably have a pretty good idea based on my earlier discussion of macronutrients, nutrigenomics, and the gut microbiome. Just to reiterate: What's good for the brain is good for the gut and good for the skin, too. If healthy eating based on the KetoFLEX 12/3 plan helps prevent or reverse Alzheimer's disease AND helps feed your skin right, it's truly something to get excited about. You'll age better, live longer while free from disease and disability, and when you look in the mirror, you'll like what you see.

Caloric restriction (CR) can positively alter the trajectory of age-related diseases and retard biological aging. Animal studies involving significant calorie restriction—between 10 and 50% fewer calories—resulted in demonstrably longer lifespans.[44] Humans are less suited to these types of strict CR studies for obvious reasons, although similar results can be inferred from animal models and intermittent fasting studies involving human subjects.[45]

Unfortunately, the effects of any modified eating strategy on skin aging are not well understood. This is the result of poor-quality studies and mixed findings. The promising news is, however, that CR in its various forms is believed to have great potential for skin rejuvenation and treatment of skin disorders.[46] One area you'll want to pay attention to in the future is wound healing efficiency. Preliminary research suggests that a 24-hour fast twice weekly after a wound injury results in quicker closing of the wound, better regeneration of the epidermal and dermal skin layers, and reduced scar formation.[47] Results were more substantial if the fasting was done *before* the injury, which may have positive implications for moderately invasive dermal procedures and/or cosmetic surgery. Stay tuned!

A WORD OF CAUTION

While intermittent, short-term fasting is generally considered safe, individuals with any type of medical condition should consult their primary care physician for advice and guidance. For some people, too much caloric restriction and fasting can decrease their baseline metabolism as well as cause them to lose muscle mass. Monitoring the ratio of muscle/fat, either with body impedance (i.e., inbodyusa.com) or a DEXA scan, can alert you to unhealthy changes in these ratios.

A lot has changed with regards to nutrition education since you (depending on your age) or I was in school. The fact that information is fluid means that by the time I finish writing this book, new knowledge will have been generated and someone will come along with a new approach to skin care. Yet, even so, it takes an average of 17 years for scientific discovery to be incorporated into clinical practice.[48] Does that mean that *Feed Your Skin Right* is 17 years ahead, 17 years behind, or somewhere in between? Let's just say, it's the truth as we know it today (tomorrow may be different). The consensus among experts is that your daily diet or eating style is a significant determinant of youthful looking skin.

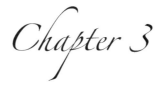

Chapter 3

THE POWER OF PLANT-BASED EATING FOR SKIN BEAUTY

Plants take the full brunt of the sun's rays every day. The purpose of many of the 5,000 antioxidant phytochemicals in the plants is protection from solar damage. You gain that protection when you ingest these substances. While scientists have isolated, extracted or synthesized individual substances, you will always be best served by eating plants of many colors and supplementing when necessary. For example, one such plant extract—*Polypodium leucotomos,* a species of fern—had high safety and efficacy for reducing the damaging effects of UV radiation. Study participants who took an oral extract for 2 months had fewer sunburns and a greater tolerance in both exposure time and UV intensity before sunburn occurred.[49]

Oral antioxidants are great for UV protection, yet they can't compete with a quality topical sunblock. Although there's no hard and fast rule, you might think of a high-antioxidant diet as providing an SPF of 3-4, versus a commercial sunblock providing an SPF of 15-50.

Phytonutrients are Your BFFs

Brightly colored vegetables, fruits, nuts, seeds, and herbs should also take up the most space on your dinner plate (at least half). We all know this is what we're supposed to do, but knowing that it's fundamental to beautiful skin makes you more likely to "eat healthy."

NOTE: You'll often see the terms "phytonutrients" and "phytochemicals" used interchangeably. It's the "chemical" part that characterizes these natural compounds which provide the rich color and aroma to whole plant foods. I prefer using "phytonutrients" when discussing how to feed your skin right. It reminds readers that these are completely natural compounds that the plants themselves utilize for their own protection against UV rays, free radicals, pathogens, and parasites.

In the past, vitamins and minerals took center stage, and although these are still important, it's the cornucopia of polyphenols and antioxidants that have achieved rockstar status, thanks to advancements in nutrition and skincare science. Phytonutrients have a valuable role in overall health and beauty, yet unlike with major micronutrients such as vitamin C or vitamin A, you won't experience a serious deficiency if you don't get enough phytonutrients in your daily diet. But the extra benefits of consuming phytonutrient-rich foods will make you re-think your eating habits. So, let's take a deep dive into why we need phytonutrients if we want young, healthy-looking skin.

BENEFITS OF PHYTONUTRIENTS
- Slow down the growth of cancer cells
- Protect against oxidative stress and reactive oxygen species (ROS)
- Reduce inflammation
- Prevent DNA damage
- Induce apoptosis (cell death) in damaged/diseased cells

You're probably more familiar with the common name for reactive oxygen species (ROS)—"free radicals"—and no, they aren't leftover hippies from the 1960s but rather, nasty little molecules that cause all types of cellular damage. ROS naturally have an unpaired electron, and they desperately want another electron. So, they're circulating in the body (on the hunt, so to speak) for an extra electron, and they'll steal that electron from anywhere they can, including the molecules that make up the membranes of skin cells. So, over time, ROS can cause deterioration of the collagen and elastin fibers in the skin, leading to fine lines, wrinkles, and saggy skin. Loss of hyaluronic acid leads to moisture (hydration) loss.

SKIN CELL DAMAGE CAUSED BY FREE RADICALS (ROS)
- Damage the DNA in the skin cells
- Damage cell membranes by stealing electrons
- Degrade collagen, elastin, and hyaluronic acid in skin
- Decrease collagen production
- Cause inflammation

FORMATION OF FREE RADICALS

- UV LIGHT
- AIR POLLUTION
- IONIZING RADIATION
- DNA DAMAGE
- INFLAMMATION
- METABOLISM
- SMOKING

Antioxidants to the Rescue!

Antioxidants donate extra electrons so that the ROS don't have to steal them. By effectively neutralizing the ROS, antioxidants prevent cellular damage. Unfortunately, one of two things—or both—can happen which accelerate skin aging. First, environmental factors such as pollution, UV exposure, ionizing radiation, chemicals, and toxins, as well as lifestyle factors such as smoking, stress, lack of sleep, and poor nutrition can produce excessive amounts of ROS; the native antioxidants in the human body simply can't keep up with demand. Second, as we get older and our environmental exposure accumulates, the native antioxidant levels decrease; there's fewer antioxidants to take care of the growing demand. Replenishing the body's antioxidant capacity is therefore critical, if you want to continue to have healthy skin beyond your 20s and 30s. Thankfully, dietary antioxidants can help your body meet this demand. One very important group of phytonutrients is the polyphenols, a type of antioxidant whose primary benefit is protecting the body's cells from free radical damage. Much of this free-radical fighting helps shield the skin from ultraviolet light and other environmental stressors like pollution. By reducing the amount of oxidative stress, inflammation is also reduced.

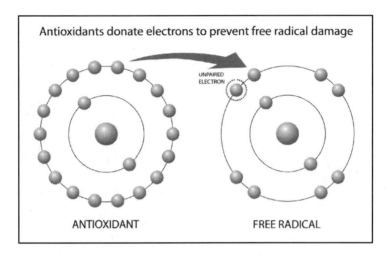

Polyphenols can be subdivided into 4 main types—flavonoids, phenolic acids, stilbenes, and lignans.[50] Flavonoid subclasses include flavonols, flavones, isoflavones, flavanones, anthocyanidins, and flavanols—I give you this not to get too much into the science, but because you've probably heard these in reference to the marketing of specific foods.

POLYPHENOLS IN COMMON PLANT-BASED FOODS

- **Flavonols** (quercetin, rutin) – asparagus, buckwheat, citrus fruits, apples, peaches, green tea
- **Flavones** – celery, red peppers, chamomile, mint, parsley, rosemary, oregano, traditional Chinese herbs, ginkgo biloba
- **Isoflavones** – soybeans, soymilk
- **Flavanones** – lemons, limes, oranges, grapefruit
- **Anthocyanidins** – blueberries, cranberries, raspberries, red and black grapes, red cabbage
- **Flavanols** – apples, red wine, green tea, dark chocolate, unsweetened cocoa powder
- **Phenolic Acid** (ellagic acid, a tannin) –cranberries, grapes, peaches, pomegranates, raspberries, strawberries, pecans, walnuts
- **Stilbenes** (resveratrol) – red wine

Polyphenols are the most abundant source of antioxidants in the human diet, so if you eat a healthy, rainbow-colored diet, your skin will really appreciate it. Currently, there are no RDAs (Recommended Dietary Allowances) for phytonutrient-rich foods, but what most nutrition experts recommend is a minimum of 5 servings; setting your goal at 8-10 servings every day is even better. The chart below shows roughly equivalent amounts making up one serving.[51]

Since foods vary in the type of phytonutrients they contain, *diversity* of the plant foods you consume is perhaps more important than simply quantity. Eat the rainbow—deep blue and purples, vibrant greens, and bright yellows and oranges, and robust reds. And, aim for organic or homegrown whenever possible.

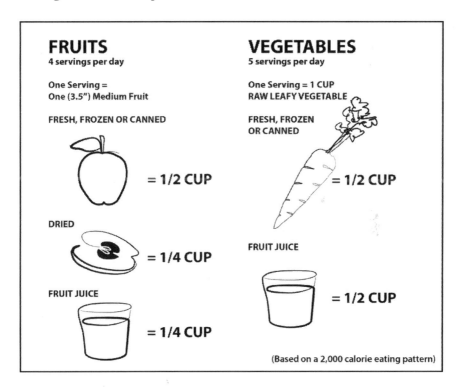

OTHER PLANT-BASED NUTRIENTS FOR HEALTHY SKIN

Carotenoids—a group of red, orange, and yellow pigments found in plant foods that have potent antioxidant capacity. In addition to protecting all cells (and particularly skin cells against oxidative stress), carotenoids facilitate cellular communication; scientists believe that this "talking" between cells might be the reason that carotenoids offer protection against cancer, specifically some forms of skin cancer.

More than 600 carotenoids have been identified, yet the superstar carotenoids for health relevancy are beta-carotene, lycopene, and lutein and zeaxanthin. The human body does not synthesize the vast majority of carotenoids, so we need to eat carotenoid-rich foods or take dietary supplements to take advantage of their health benefits. Dietary carotenoids are more absorbable (bioavailable) when you eat them with a good fat, such as olive oil, avocado oil, or avocado. I discuss carotenoids more in depth in PART II: What Supplements Should I Take?

FOODS RICH IN BETA-CAROTENE	• Sweet potatoes • Carrots • Pumpkins • Butternut squash • Cantaloupes • Mangoes • Peaches	• Apricots • Spinach • Kale • Romaine lettuce • Broccoli • Turnips
FOODS RICH IN LYCOPENE	• Sun-dried tomatoes • Tomatoes (cooked) • Guavas • Watermelon • Tomatoes (uncooked) • Pink Grapefruits • Red peppers (cooked)	• Papayas • Fuyu Persimmons • Mangoes • Asparagus • Apricots • Peaches
FOODS RICH IN LUTEIN/ ZEAXANTHIN	• Spinach (cooked) • Kale (cooked) • Swiss chard (cooked) • Collard greens (cooked) • Green peas • Summer squash • Pumpkin	• Broccoli • Brussels sprouts • Asparagus • Romaine lettuce • Carrots • Pistachios

- **Beta-carotene**—the body converts this phytonutrient into vitamin A; this is why beta-carotene is sometimes referred to as provitamin A. Vitamin A helps prevent skin damage caused by UV exposure, pollution, and smoking. It also enhances collagen production for overall healthier skin and wound healing.
- **Lycopene**—this carotenoid is probably best known for its prostate benefits, but it also has benefits for healthy-aging skin. Lycopene increases the body's production of procollagen, a precursor to collagen, which in turn, helps lessen UV skin damage.
- **Lutein & Zeaxanthin**—this carotenoid duo is likely more familiar for protecting the eyes against UV and blue light, but it's also good for skin health. Regular intake improves skin tone, protects against photoaging, and reduces the risk of developing skin cancer.

Vitamin C—an antioxidant powerhouse which also supports collagen formation. L-ascorbic acid is the functional form of vitamin C which is necessary for various biological reactions within the body. Ascorbic acid is an electron donor for enzymes which help stabilize the structure of collagen and synthesize carnitine (required for energy), amino acids, and various hormones. Vitamin C helps reduce skin inflammation by neutralizing free radicals and assists with fine lines and firmer skin. The human body cannot manufacture its own vitamin C, so you must get it from foods or supplements. Because only a limited amount of oral vitamin C is able to reach the skin, topical application is advantageous. Of course, vitamin C-rich foods should be incorporated into a wellness-based diet, especially if you have the *GSTT1* genetic variant which can result in an increased need for vitamin C.

FOODS RICH IN VITAMIN C

- Black currants
- Kiwifruit
- Green bell peppers
- Strawberries
- Broccoli
- Pineapples
- Lemons
- Honeydew
- Red peppers
- Guavas
- Oranges
- Papayas
- Kale
- Brussels sprouts
- Grapefruit

Ceramides—a type of lipid (fat) found in the skin whose function it is to help prevent moisture loss from the skin. In other words, ceramides are important for hydrated skin; without adequate levels in the skin, your skin can become dry and flaky. Ceramides are found in both plant-based and animal foods.

PLANT-BASED CERAMIDES
• Whole-grain wheat
• Wheat germ
• Millet
• Brown rice
• Sweet potato
• Spinach
• Soybeans

Don't Forget the Fiber

Eating lots of fiber doesn't just keep you from getting constipated. It feeds and nurtures the beneficial gut bacteria which in turn, supports the gut-brain-skin axis. Of course, when you eat a diet that emphasizes plant-based foods, you naturally get a lot of fiber, along with all those wonderful phytonutrients. Be sure to drink enough water—at least two liters a day—to keep your bowels moving smoothly and comfortably, and your skin hydrated.

HIGH FIBER VEGETABLES	HIGH FIBER FRUITS
• Green peas	• Raspberries
• Broccoli	• Blackberries
• Turnip greens	• Pears
• Brussels sprouts	• Apples (unpeeled)
• Cauliflower	• Banana
• Carrots	• Orange
• Artichoke hearts	• Strawberries
HIGH FIBER LEGUMES	**HIGH FIBER NUTS & SEEDS**
• Split peas	• Chia seeds
• Chickpeas	• Flax seeds
• Pigeon peas	• Sunflower seeds
• Lentils	• Almonds
• Lima beans	• Pistachios
• Black beans	

Plant-Based Food is Your Best Protection

Unless you have a genetic variant that predisposes you to a specific vitamin deficiency, most, if not all of your micronutrient needs can be met with a varied, healthy diet that is primarily comprised of minimally-processed plant-based foods. If you have a diagnosed skin condition, such as rosacea, which is worsened by a specific plant-based food(s), avoid that food(s). There are plenty of other phytonutrient superstars just waiting for you to eat them. I recommend you shop the entire produce section, not just what you normally frequent. Shop your local farmers market or a neighborhood ethnic market to try something new. If you live near the woods, join a foraging club to discover a bounty of edible plants, including wild mushrooms and herbs.

We're only now beginning to scratch the surface of understanding what the thousands of phytonutrients do to protect plants, let alone protect and improve human health and skin beauty. As this field of study evolves, we are sure to learn even more. In the meantime, be adventurous in your quest for those 5,000+ phytonutrients.

Chapter 4

HOW YOUR GUT-BRAIN-SKIN ARE ALL CONNECTED

No doubt that you've probably heard of the "gut microbiome," "dysbiosis," "gut-brain-skin axis," and "leaky gut," as these terms have made their way into our common vocabulary and are no longer exclusively used by the scientific and medical community. Many of these terms are associated with over-the-counter supplements (i.e., probiotics, prebiotics) and other nutrition-based products that are designed to promote GI health and/or improve our bloating or pooping problems. Before we move ahead, I'll define the basic terminology.

- **Gut Microbiome** (includes "gut bugs," "gut microbes," or "gut microbiota")—the ecosystem inhabiting the gastrointestinal tract; it is home to trillions of bacteria, viruses, fungi, and archaea (single-celled organisms) which live together in symbiotic relationships.

- **Dysbiosis**—the imbalance among the gut bugs, generally recognized as too much "bad" bacteria and too little "good" bacteria; this imbalance is believed to contribute to specific conditions and/or diseases of the body, including the brain and skin.

- **Gut-Brain-Skin Axis**—this relational theory suggests that the gut microbiome, the brain, and the skin interact via nerve and chemical signals to influence one another's health.

- **Leaky Gut**—often referred to as excessive intestinal permeability, this condition occurs when the tight junctions between the cells of the gut wall become weakened or loose. This allows ingested toxins, incompletely digested food proteins, and some harmful fragments of the gut bugs to enter the bloodstream where the immune system attacks them by initiating inflammation that can then run rampant throughout the body.

The Gut Microbiome

The gut microbiome is comprised primarily of bacteria, and today, more is known about the bacteria and what they do than is the case with any of the other microbes. Each individual has between 300 and 1,000 different species of bacteria, and about 30-40 species contribute 99% of the bacteria in the microbiome. Individuals' microbiomes are unique; no two people have the same composition or distribution of microbiota.

In 2019, researchers at MIT published a paper identifying 7,758 different strains of microbes isolated from 90 different people.[52] Microbiome analysis is commercially available if you're curious as to which strains inhabit your GI tract, but the key take-away is *diversity*—the presence of many different strains. This appears to be an important determinant of health. I will occasionally return to the concept of microbiota diversity and the role plant-based nutrition plays in both preserving it and increasing it.

If we think about the microbiome in its entirety, it's considered to be an organ like the heart, liver, or kidneys, and as such it warrants attention and care. The combination of bacteria, viruses, and fungi collectively weigh between 3.5-4.5 pounds, about the same weight as your brain. Optimized feeding of the microbiome—and other positive lifestyle habits—contributes to a variety of health benefits. It's a reciprocal relationship. Certain bacteria aid in digestion and synthesize B vitamins, while others synthesize neurotransmitters, including serotonin. In fact, about 95% of all serotonin, the neurotransmitter responsible for happiness, is produced in the gut. This connection between the gut and brain is known as the gut-brain axis. If your brain is not happy, you will not radiate beauty, no matter what aesthetic procedures you undergo, or topicals you may apply.

While there is no evidence that the neurotransmitters produced by the gut bacteria directly cross the blood-brain barrier, they do influence the signals sent to the brain via the vagus nerve. Furthermore, this axis plays an important role in skin health. Those same neurotransmitters secreted by the gut microbiome find their way into circulation and into the skin—a healthy gut equals healthy skin.

MOOD-ALTERING NEUROTRANSMITTERS	
GABA	
• Critical to the proper functioning of the brain and nervous system. • Produces a calming effect by slowing down neural activity.	Produced by • *Lactobacillus* • *Bifidobacterium*
NOREPINEPHRINE	
• Plays an important role in wakefulness, mood, mental focus, and memory storage. • Increases heart rate, blood pressure, blood flow to skeletal muscle, and release of stored glucose, while decreasing blood flow to the GI tract and slowing of GI motility – fight-or-flight response.	Produced by • *Escherichia* • *Bacillus* • *Saccharomyces*
ACETYLCHOLINE	
• Plays a role in mental focus, learning, and memorization of information. • Assists with sleep and arousal, skeletal muscle contractions, and stimulates the release of serotonin and dopamine (the "feel good" brain chemicals).	Produced by • *Lactobacillus*
SEROTONIN	
• Stabilizes mood and encourages feelings of happiness and well-being to stave off depression. • Affects sleep cycles and influences appetite, metabolism and digestion.	Produced by • *Candida* • *Streptococcus* • *Escherichia* • *Enterococcus*

THE POWER OF PREBIOTICS

Prebiotics are the fiber-dense foods that provide nourishment for the beneficial gut bacteria and help them thrive; as a result, the populations of these good gut bacteria increase. Healthy prebiotic foods include onions, garlic, leeks, asparagus, Jerusalem artichokes, and bananas. Prebiotics are also available in supplement form—made from the processed fiber of fresh food sources. For example, inulin, the natural soluble fiber found in many plants, can be modified and added back into other food products—often those foods that are already high in sugar such as granola or protein bars. I advocate getting prebiotics from whole foods whenever possible.

When I began my nutrition education way back in the 1970s, there wasn't a lot known about the gut microbiome, much less that it actually existed. The general consensus was that the stalks, stems, and more pithy parts of edible plants were just "roughage," devoid of any real nutritional value except for the anti-constipation benefit. The real value we believed was in the top, green leafy parts of vegetables, but like most things, we're getting smarter all the time—and thank goodness, now we appreciate the entire plant!

When we consume fibrous plants—a.k.a. roughage—the microbes in the intestine feed off of and ferment these indigestible carbohydrates, and in doing so, produce short-chain fatty acids (SCFAs). Aside from supplying about 5-10% of the body's energy needs, SCFAs have many important functions within the body with respect to countering disease. They provide anti-inflammatory, anticarcinogenic, and antimicrobial benefits which contribute to gut and immune balance.[53] One particular SCFA, butyric acid (butyrate), provides energy for the epithelial (skin) cells in the colon, which is one of the reasons why experts recommend a high-fiber diet for the prevention of colon cancer. Another SCFA, propionate, is also produced by the bacteria in the colon. Propionate circulates widely in the bloodstream and reaches the skin where it has anti-inflammatory actions.[54]

The influence of SCFAs isn't confined to just the gut microbiome or the larger, more expansive digestive tract. Researchers speculate that SCFAs play an important role in the gut-brain communication.[55] The skin is also happy with this anti-inflammatory powerhouse because when inflammation is under control and the gut-brain-skin axis is balanced, your skin glows naturally. Eating more roughage is an easy and relatively inexpensive nutritional choice for improving skin health. Additionally, research shows that inflamed skin cells respond to topical application of butyrate, which may prove helpful in inflammatory skin conditions.[56]

Before the Prebiotics, There Were the Probiotics

Probiotics is a synonym for beneficial bacteria, and it encompasses the bacteria strains that have been researched and shown to support gut and immune health. Probiotics are typically found in foods that have been naturally fermented (but not pasteurized), such as sauerkraut, kimchi, tempeh, miso, kombucha (watch the sugar content!), pickles (without benzoate as a preservative), kefir, traditional buttermilk, and yogurt (stay away from the sugar-added varieties). Supplemental probiotics may be more convenient for some people, and in this case, I recommend a quality product with a high CFU (colony forming units) count and the presence of many different strains—for the diversity factor. I have a few favorites.

- I am a fan of Microbiome Labs' (microbiomelabs.com) product—SereneSkin™. It contains a mixture of *Bacillus* species along with Vitamin K2. The combination product helps fight free radical damage, support digestion and immune function, balance the gut microbiome and maintain collagen for skin firmness and thickness. There is increasing research on the role K2 plays in skin health and beauty. SereneSkin has been shown to increase propionate, the key SCFA which reaches the skin.

- Dermala's SUPPLEMEANT to Be® (dermala.com) has a robust mix of minerals, vitamins, six probiotics (including *Lactobacillus rhamnosus*) and spinach leaf extract. The product has good clinical results on acne improvement. Dermala was hatched up at the University of California San Diego working with Johnson & Johnson's Innovation Incubator, so the science is solid.

- HUM Skin Squad Pre+Probiotic™ (humnutrition.com). I don't have personal experience with this product, but it has a good mix of prebiotic species and features Konjac root, also known as glucomannan. This herb grows in parts of Asia, and it's loaded with soluble dietary fiber.

- Garden of Life Skin+. Garden of Life (gardenoflife.com) is one of the direct-to-consumer nutraceutical companies that emphasizes quality and safety in its ingredients. Their formulation contains 90 billion CFU and 12 probiotic strains, along with Vitamin A and lycopene (an important antioxidant, usually derived from tomatoes).

A healthy microbiome balance is approximately 80% good bacteria to 20% bad bacteria, but if the bad bacteria start replicating without restraint, the microbiome suffers and the result may be some type of infection or illness. For example, small intestinal bacterial overgrowth (SIBO) occurs when certain bacteria not native to the small intestine colonize too greatly, leading to a whole host of medical problems including malabsorption of vitamins and nutrients, electrolyte imbalance, anemia, diarrhea, weight loss, and osteoporosis.

A condition similar to SIBO is small intestinal fungal overgrowth (SIFO), which includes candidiasis. Yeast (candida) overgrowth commonly causes GI symptoms in immunocompromised patients or those taking antibiotics or steroids, but may be under-diagnosed in seemingly healthy people. Symptoms include belching, indigestion, bloating, nausea, diarrhea, and flatulence.

If we agree that SIBO and SIFO result from dysbiosis in the small intestine, we should also recognize what the "bad" bacteria and fungus like to eat—refined carbohydrates. If your gut bacteria and yeast are screaming "Feed me sugar," and you oblige them, you're allowing them to proliferate further and in doing so, undermining your skin's health and appearance.

Unless you are a long-term, mostly plant-based, organic eater who was born vaginally and has never taken oral antibiotics, there's a chance that your microbiome has been compromised to some degree. Microbial analysis is one way to get a baseline of which specific bacteria strains are actually inhabiting your gut. Companies such as Viome (viome.com), Sun Genomics (floré.com) and BiomeFx (biomefx.com) offer in-home microbiome testing; you provide a stool sample, mail it back, and receive a detailed list of bacteria with dietary suggestions to improve diversity. Both Viome and Floré link the test results to purchasing recommendations for their probiotics. The advantage of the BiomeFx test is that it utilizes whole genome sequencing; the entire genetic spectrum of the bacteria is profiled, rather than just a narrow snapshot. This provides a much more detailed analysis upon which recommendations can be made. Currently the BiomeFx test is only available through practitioners.

Whole genome microbiome sequencing, as shown in this sample BiomeFx report, provides detailed and specific information your practitioner can use to help personalize your treatment.

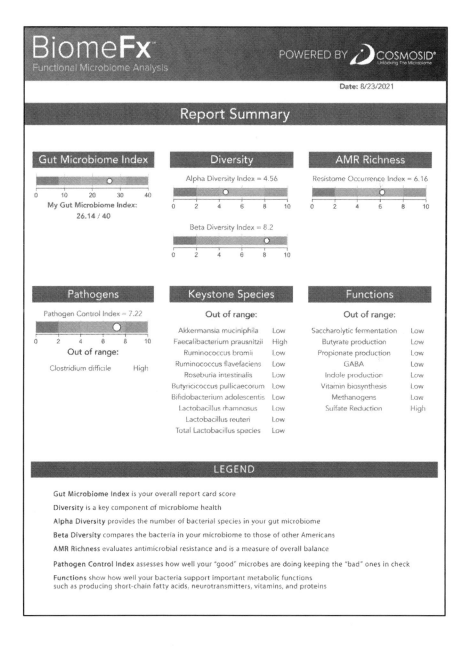

Microbiome Antagonists

A number of commonly prescribed medications can negatively impact the microbiome. Oral antibiotics can have a devastating effect. It's the job of these drugs to destroy bacteria, which can be a lifesaver—when destruction of dangerous bacteria is medically necessary. Following a course of antibiotics, building back the microbiome with probiotic foods and healthy eating strategies can help. Research suggests that just one round of antibiotics may affect the microbiome for a year or longer.[57] Most wellness-oriented physicians will prescribe probiotics along with antibiotics, to be used during and well after the antibiotics have run their course.

Three additional types of drugs which may antagonize the gut bacteria include anti-acid proton-pump inhibitors prescribed for reflux, metformin for type 2 diabetes, and laxatives.[58] If you regularly take these medications, discuss with your physician or nutrition professional how, with an improved lifestyle and diet program, you can decrease or eliminate their use.

Another microbiome disrupter is chronic, unresolved psychological stress. It can affect the gut microbiome because of the bi-directional connection between the gut and the brain (the gut-brain axis). Studies of animals experiencing chronic exposure to psychological stress had significant changes to their intestinal microbiota, leading to imbalance and loss of diversity.[59] When it comes to optimal mental health, preserving the good gut bacteria responsible for producing key neurotransmitters is important. Avoiding stress entirely may be difficult, but learning ways to manage stress and to more efficiently allocate time and resources will help.

The diagram on the next page shows the bidirectional connection between the gut and the brain. When the brain is under stress, it signals the body to produce more cortisol. It also ramps up the sympathetic nervous system, getting the body ready to fight or flee. This activation also disrupts the gut microbiome as well as the normal healthy motility of the intestines. The brain, on the other hand, constantly receives nervous signals from the gut microbiome via the vagus nerve.

One of the emerging therapeutic areas for gut and brain health revolves around non-invasively stimulating the parasympathetic nervous system to counterbalance excess sympathetic stress. GammaCore (gammacore.com) is a hand-held vagus nerve stimulating device that when gently pressed to the neck increases parasympathetic stimulation, calming the brain and gut. The device has multiple FDA clearances, most notably for migraine and cluster headache prevention and treatment. It has been designed to be used at home, 8-12 minutes a day.

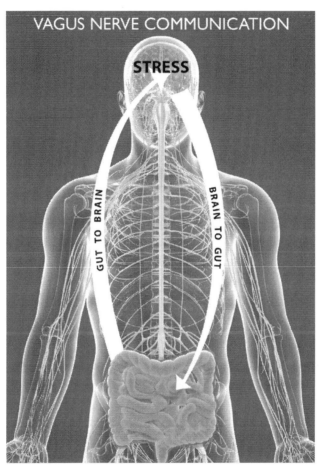

LEAKY GUT—LEAKY SKIN

Your gut is lined by epithelial cells that separate "you" from "non-you." This lining is only one cell thick. Ideally the nutrients from foods should be absorbed by the gut cells directly into the bloodstream. When the GI tract is leaky at one or multiple locations, undigested food proteins, environmental toxins (i.e., pesticides) and even harmful microbes from the gut microbiome (Think: food poisoning.) can gain access to the body where they go on to wreak havoc. It's like letting a group of thieves in through the front door of your home so they can ransack whatever they find; some go upstairs (your brain); some go to the kitchen (your joints); some go to the family room (your organs); and some go to all the bedrooms (your skin). Of course, the ransacking triggers a silent alarm (your immune system) and the police (your immune cells) are dispatched with guns drawn and handcuffs ready! If the police get into a gun battle with the invaders, this can cause even more damage.

A healthy immune system recognizes that these substances are foreign to the body and mounts an effective inflammatory response to destroy them. However, when leaky gut becomes pervasive, the inflammation becomes chronic. It may subside, but it never really goes away and is said to be systemic, low-grade inflammation. The body itself is unable to return to a state of homeostasis, and years or decades of leaky gut may eventually contribute to food sensitivities and autoimmune diseases which affect organs and tissues, including the brain and skin.

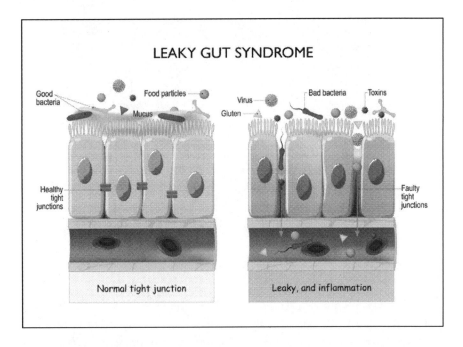

Both the gut and skin share some common anatomical features which position them as barrier and immune-regulating organs. Some permeability through the skin's epithelial cells is good, as it allows topically applied nutrients to be absorbed. Yet, if the permeability becomes excessive and allows the wrong substances to enter, then it is considered "leaky skin."

Dermatology researchers measure this leakiness by seeing how much water gets lost through the skin. When the skin barrier is not functioning well, excess water is lost and the skin takes on a more shriveled appearance. Many of the topicals work by providing barrier protection to reduce water loss from the skin.

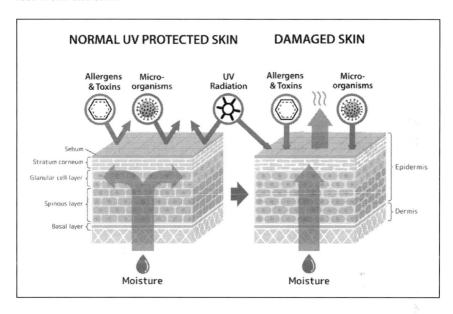

How Do You Know if Your Gut is Leaky?

At present, the best measure of leaky gut is measuring stool zonulin, a protein which controls permeability of the tight junctions in the GI lining. Zonulin can also be more easily measured in the blood, but because other organs also produce this protein, the measurement might not be as reflective of pure GI issues. Tight junctions are part of the precisely regulated system which allows nutrients from ingested food to cross from the GI tract into the bloodstream. When the system is functioning properly, zonulin concentrations are normal, but when it malfunctions (i.e., becomes leaky), zonulin levels increase. Alessio Fasano, MD and his research team at the University of Maryland School of Medicine discovered zonulin in 2000, later calling it the "biological door to inflammation, autoimmunity, and cancer."[60]

It was Dr. Fasano's early research into celiac disease and type 1 diabetes that led to the discovery of zonulin. In his decades of research, Dr. Fasano discovered that gluten activates zonulin, which means that eating gluten could trigger this dangerous cascade in genetically predisposed individuals.

Renowned neurologist David Perlmutter, MD also cautions against a gluten-laden diet for its impact on cognitive health. In one of Dr. Perlmutter's many books—*Grain Brain*—he describes how utilizing healthy fats as the primary fuel source, instead of carbs, boosts the brain's ability to function and helps defend against cognitive decline and/or neurological diseases. We already know that healthy, plant-based fats are good for younger-looking skin, so eating more of them (and going gluten-free), is perhaps helping to keep our brains young, too.

Celiac disease is characterized by small intestinal lining damage and malabsorption of some nutrients which is caused by the immune system's reaction to gluten. Celiac disease can be quite debilitating with continued gluten consumption; the intestinal damage leads to bloating, abdominal pain, nausea and vomiting, constipation, diarrhea, weight loss, anemia, fatigue, and nutrient deficiencies. In children, celiac disease may result in abnormal growth and development. Adults may develop osteoporosis, osteomalacia (soft bones), joint pain, dermatitis, mouth ulcers, headaches, nervous system injury, balance problems, and cognitive impairment. These seemingly non-GI related conditions are, once again, tied to the gut-brain-skin axis and thus again demonstrate the importance of avoiding the triggers that compromise overall gut health.

Celiac and type 1 diabetes are just two of more than 80 recognized autoimmune diseases, and although the research has not proven that leaky gut causes these conditions, it certainly suggests that leaky gut and other biological malfunctions occur at the same time.[61] So, if you have already been diagnosed with an autoimmune disease or an autoimmune inflammatory skin condition such as psoriasis, eczema, or scleroderma,[62,63,64] there's a strong possibility that you also have leaky gut. Even if you do not have a diagnosed disease, many believe that gut antagonists are so pervasive in the modern world, that no one is really immune.

The Brain's Point of View
Now, switching gears a little. *What does your brain think about all this?* Well, the brain itself can be an influential, but less understood, gut offender by

virtue of its physical connection, which isn't simply unidirectional (gut→brain). Communication via the vagus nerve is bidirectional (gut→←brain), which means brain health is just as likely to influence gut health and vice versa. The vagus nerve is the tenth cranial nerve which interfaces with the heart, lungs, and digestive tract. Emotions such as anxiety, stress, and depression affect the gut microbiota and alter their activity. This is the rationale behind the notion of "it's a gut feeling," or "I feel it in my gut."

Negative changes to the gut microbiome may then send negative signals to the skin microbiome which in turn, trigger a flare-up of acne or psoriasis. Essentially, the brain acts as the perpetrator of bad skin by inducing changes in the gut. In this instance, perhaps it's more accurate to say brain-gut-skin axis.

3-STEP APPROACH TO IMPROVING THE GUT MICROBIOME FOR BETTER SKIN HEALTH

Tackling skin health from the inside out requires a three-part approach to supporting the gut lining and the gut microbiome—Remove, Repair, Replace/repopulate.

STEP #1 – REMOVE THE GUT OFFENDERS
Protecting the integrity of the delicate lining of the GI tract is an imperative. Here's a concise refresher on what you should avoid whenever possible:
- Processed foods
- Fast foods
- Refined cooking oils
- High glycemic index foods
- Artificial sweeteners
- Gluten (for celiac disease or gluten sensitivity)
- GMO foods
- Pesticide/herbicide-contaminated foods (most notably glyphosate)
- Synthetic/chemical food additives
- Excessive alcohol
- Excessive caffeine
- Unnecessary use of oral antibiotics
- Pain medications (NSAIDs, ibuprofen, opioids)

- Gut-irritating medications (proton pump inhibitors for acid reflux, metformin for type 2 diabetes, laxatives.)[65]
- Chronic, unresolved stress
- Smoking
- Lack of sleep

STEP #2 – REPAIR THE GI LINING

The repair phase is an ongoing (lifetime) process. Once the gut offenders are removed, inflammation subsides and the GI lining begins repairing itself, yet for as good as the human body is at self-repair, frequently it's not enough. You can employ targeted nutrition to improve the GI lining and maintain its integrity. Here's where I look to Marvin Singh, MD, an integrative gastroenterologist in San Diego, California. Dr. Singh has researched the most effective and accessible nutrition supplements, medical foods, and herbal teas, and utilizes them in his Precisione Medicine Clinic (precisionclinic.com). His gut-reinforcing recommendations include:

- **Serum-derived bovine (cow) immunoglobulin** (SBI) – a medical food prescribed and monitored by a doctor. SBI is a concentrated formula of immunoglobulins (>50% IgG, 1% IgA, and 5% IgM), albumin and other proteins which helps manage chronic diarrhea or frequent, loose stools. The immunoglobulins bind to and eliminate pathogenic microbes which helps restore homeostasis within the intestines. Restoration of normal GI function and nutrient absorption promotes normal bowel movements. MegaIgG2000 from Microbiome Labs is one such product.

- **Bovine (cow) or goat colostrum** – a nutritional supplement made from whole colostrum which contains a high percentage of immunoglobulins, immune bioactives, and growth factors. Colostrum helps neutralize gut pathogens, feed the microbiome, repair GI lining damage, reduce inflammation, increase nutrient absorption, and stimulate growth of lean body mass.[66] Because bovine colostrum has been clinically shown to improve leaky gut caused by NSAID use,[67] I also highly recommend it. Colostrum-LD® from Sovereign Laboratories is my preferred brand.

- **L-glutamine** – an amino acid supplement. Glutamine plays a role in maintaining a strong intestinal lining and is synthesized naturally by the body. In times of stress, glutamine demand increases and must be obtained from foods or supplements. Food sources include beef, chicken, fish, eggs, dairy products, beans, beets, Brussels sprouts, cabbage, carrots, celery, kale, papaya, parsley, spinach, and miso. Supplemental glutamine has shown positive results during high intensity exercise[68] and critical illness,[69] two situations which increase intestinal permeability.

- **Zinc L-carnosine (ZnC)** – a dietary supplement and a drug (polaprezinc). Zinc carnosine stimulates mucus production, maintains integrity of the GI lining, and neutralizes free radicals. As a drug, zinc carnosine treats gastric ulcers by accelerating GI wound healing. As a supplement, ZnC helps prevent leaky gut and research has shown it works well with bovine colostrum,[70] thus making it a key nutrient for skin beauty.

- **Spore probiotic with *Saccharomyces boulardii*** – Spore-based probiotics contain beneficial bacteria from the soil. Because the spores are encapsulated, they survive the harsh acid of our stomachs. *S. boulardii* is a beneficial species of yeast and offers protection against small and large intestine bacterial pathogens that cause dysbiosis and diarrhea. My preferred brands are MegaSporeBiotic™ from Microbiome Labs (microbiomelabs.com) and ProBioSpore from Designs for Health (available online).

- **Herbal teas (cumin, coriander, and fennel)** – an ancient Ayurvedic remedy for digestive problems. Herbal teas offer soothing relaxation, help calm an irritated gut, relieve bloating and gas, and balance blood glucose.

Because strengthening the gut lining is key to preventing leaky gut and improving skin health, many of the nutritional supplements that I discuss in PART II contain some of these ingredients.

STEP #3 – REPLACE/REPOPULATE THE MICROBIOTA

Once these microbiome antagonists are removed, your focus should be on tilting the scale in favor of the good bacteria (probiotics). Through the introduction of oral probiotics, skin conditions such as acne, atopic dermatitis, and photoaging can be improved.[71,72,73] This is also a good strategy for women who have developed a vaginal yeast infection after a round of antibiotics.

The replace & repopulate phase can take place in tandem with the repair phase. Research has identified specific bacterial strains that are associated with various skin conditions. In this case, your dermatologist may recommend supplementing with the probiotic that most directly impacts your skin problem.

CONDITION	PREBIOTICS	PROBIOTICS
ACNE	Gucomannan	Lactobacillus Bifidobacterium Enterococcus
PSORIASIS	Butyrate	Saccharomyces Bifidobacterium Lactobacillus
ALLERGIC CONTACT DERMATITIS	Fructooligosaccharides	Lactobacillus Bifidobacterium E. Coli
PHOTOAGING	Galactooligosaccharides	Lactobacillus Bifidobacterium
WOUNDS		Kefir Saccharomyces Lactobacillus

The combined use of prebiotic and probiotic foods and supplements can help address skin conditions by positively impacting the skin microbiome. In general, *Lactobacillus, Bifidobacterium, Lactococcus,* and oligosaccharides contribute to healthy states. Oligosccharides are short chains of plant sugars. They can consist either of fructose (fructooligosaccharides) or galactose (galactooligosaccharides). Gucomannan is a dietary fiber made from the root of the Konjac plant which comes from Asia.

THE ROLE OF PROFESSIONAL TESTING

In addition to just assessing the microbiome, clinicians who specialize in personalized nutrition have many types of panels to guide treatment. Stool tests such as GI Effects®, GI360™, and GI-Map can alert the practitioner to problems with digestive enzyme adequacy, the presence of intestinal permeability and inflammation in the gut, pathogenic bacteria, or measurement of short chain fatty acids. These tests can be very informative in personalizing the 3R Program. They have their place alongside tests like Viome or BiomeFx to individualize probiotic support.

THE SKIN MICROBIOME

Not only does the skin have its own microbiome, it takes up a lot of real estate as the largest organ in the human body. The skin and gut microbiomes do share some of the same species, such as staphylococci, streptococci, and candida; similarly, no two people have the exact same composition of bacteria, viruses, and fungi (and some mites, too) inhabiting their skin.

Although it is perhaps lesser known, the skin microbiome has become a hot topic in recent years, especially with skincare and cosmetic companies which are poised to drive the research that will validate their anti-aging products. Their aim is—through the use of topicals—to manipulate the skin's microbiome as a means of enhancing skin texture, reducing fine lines and wrinkles, and restoring that youthful glow. With an annual $135B beauty industry, it's clear there's no shortage of consumer demand.[74]

Along with the skin's seven layers, the skin microbiome provides a defensive barrier between the outside world and the muscles, ligaments, bones, and internal organs, including the gut microbiome. Researchers have identified 1000+ bacterial species, and a literal million bacteria live on a square centimeter of skin.[75] About 80 fungi species can also be found in the skin. The majority of the microorganisms reside on the skin's surface and just beneath in the top layers of the epidermis; the hair follicles, sweat glands, and sebaceous glands allow the microorganisms deeper entry into the dermis, yet relatively contained.[76] Interestingly, the skin microbiome of each person also differs depending on which part of the body is examined—the face, hands, armpits, and feet.

The make-up of any one person's skin microbiome is influenced by a variety of factors. Nutrition certainly plays a role, but so does an individual's physiology (gender, age); genotype (susceptibility genes); living environment (geography, climate); occupation or working environment; personal hygiene; immune system (inflammation, previous microbial exposure); and underlying health conditions (diabetes). The most dramatic changes in the skin microbiome occur as one transitions from childhood to puberty to adulthood. But even before that, we receive different microbes from mom depending upon whether we were born vaginally or by Cesarean section.

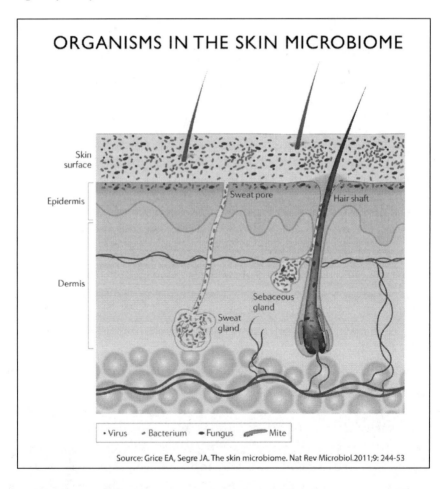

Source: Grice EA, Segre JA. The skin microbiome. Nat Rev Microbiol.2011;9: 244-53

We've long known that the buildup of sebum coupled with an accumulation of dead skin cells is the perfect breeding ground for *Propionibacterium acnes* (*P. acnes*), a type of bacteria with multiple strains that is typically associated with acne. But nearly a decade ago, there was a big 'aha' moment that emerged. Chief investigator Huiying Li, PhD, from the UCLA Microbiome Center, identified a "friendly" strain of *P. acnes* that offered protection against the "bad" acne-causing *P. acnes* strains.[77] It's similar to live probiotics ("good" bacteria) in yogurt or kefir which help protect the gut from otherwise harmful bacteria. Dr. Li's research shows us that with all the diverse bacterial species cohabitating on the skin's surface—some good, some bad—the good guys typically outnumber the bad guys and thus, protect against those microorganisms that seek to infect the skin. And again, like the gut microbiome, the more diversity of good bacterial strains the better it is for overall skin health.

This realization—that by increasing the good bacteria on the skin we could help regulate the skin's protective acid pH, strengthen its barrier function, and downregulate inflammation—has fueled an entire industry. Today, almost every major skincare company is researching the best probiotics to add to their topical products.

One of the first out of the gate to create a skin microbiome assessment report is UK based Labskin (a division of Deepverge PLC) who launched their Skin Trust Club app (skintrustclub.com) in the UK and Ireland in 2021 and later that year brought it to the US. The Skin Trust Club health tracking app provides personalized skincare suggestions based on your unique skin microbiome. You order the kit, collect your sample by simply swabbing the cheek area, and send the swab in for analysis. The team at Skin Trust Club uses a combination of advanced sequencing technologies, bioinformatics, and artificial intelligence algorithms to create your unique microbiome score. The report and personalized skincare recommendations are sent directly to your iOS or Android phone.

I'll have more to say about the skin microbiome in PART III: What Topicals Should I Apply?

Hyper-Vigilant Skin Hygiene & Loss of Bacterial Diversity

Absolutely *everything* you put on your skin will affect the skin microbiome. That means the long list of nearly unpronounceable and unrecognizable ingredients on the product label of many of your most-used products that come into contact with your skin—parabens, sulfates, silicone, dimethicones, phthalates, petrolatum, artificial colors, and fragrances. And as I mentioned earlier, the average person uses a lot of personal care products every day.

Furthermore, cleansing frequency, as well as the mechanical cleansing habits themselves (i.e., rubbing, scrubbing) we do before applying personal care products can disrupt the skin microbiome. Scrubbing or using a harsh cleanser removes the good bacteria that balances the skin microbiome and provides skin barrier protection. So, remember: It's okay to get a little dirty once in a while. As for the skin microbiome, gently cleanse your face, neck, and body—don't overdo it.

> ### HABITS THAT HELP AVOID MICROBIAL IMBALANCES
>
> - Don't overuse liquid soaps and body washes, especially those labeled "antibacterial."
>
> - Don't preferentially use antibacterial lotions and hand sanitizers, unless you're using them to mitigate a high-risk COVID-19 situation.
>
> - Don't rely on over-the-counter probiotic supplements which contain small amount of a few probiotic strains—they probably don't do much good because they're incapable of positively influencing the microbiome.

Current theory suggests that low diversity in the skin microbiome may contribute to some skin conditions, including acne, eczema, and rosacea. As a whole, our skin is cleaner than ever before; hygiene is good, but there's a possibility of being "too clean." Abrasive and harsh cleansers eliminate the good bacteria on the skin's surface, and frequent cleansing prevents these strains from regenerating. And with the loss of good bacteria, the bad bacteria remain strong and unchecked. A good old-fashioned bar of mild soap does more to preserve the skin microbiome than an antibacterial soap or hand sanitizer. So, unless you are in a potentially infectious situation (i.e., COVID-19), clean your skin as you would a baby—mild and gentle.

It's All Connected…Good Gut, Good Brain, and Great Skin
Now that you know how your gut, brain, and skin are connected, I surmise that you have a new-found understanding and appreciation of the food choices you make every day, at every meal. Suddenly, the choice between eating an apple and eating apple pie becomes significantly easier. Knowing that you thrive when your gut microbiota thrive is motivation itself, but looking into the mirror and seeing healthy, beautiful skin reflected back is truly rewarding. If you feed your skin right, you'll find yourself enveloped with glowing radiance that projects outward to others.

Chapter 5

EATING RIGHT FOR YOUR GENES

When it comes to the emerging field of nutrition and genes, I'm going to start off by inserting an adverb into my (our) favorite phrase…really.

It *really* depends.

Well, wait a minute, aren't genes locked in and we can't do anything to change them? There are some genes that are called deterministic. Early on, they determine things like hair or eye color, or worst case, a genetically inherited disease. But this is only part of the story. Our genes may be hardwired, but their expression is not. Genes influence our nutrition, and nutrition influences our genes. Both play a key role in overall health and skin appearance. Before we dive more deeply into this relationship, let's briefly review some science.

HOW GENES WORK

DNA—the double stranded helix we inherit from our parents—makes RNA, and RNA in turn creates amino acids which are the basis for proteins. This takes place in each of the 37 trillion cells of your body. The amino acids that are created are the ultimate actors, doing the work of influencing cellular reactions.

DNA consists of pairs of nucleotides linked to one another. The nucleotides are abbreviated as letters: A for Adenine, T for Thymine, G for Guanine and C for Cytosine. In DNA, the A pairs with the T, and the G with the C. You've got roughly three billion of these pairs of nucleotides in each of your cells. These three billion nucleotide pairs are arranged in about 23,000 genes. In the genetic code, each three nucleotides in a row code for a single amino acid.

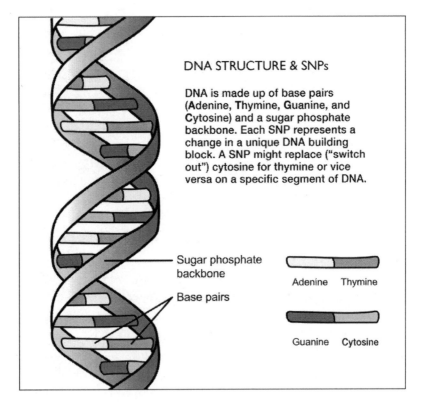

Why Your Genetics are Personal

When talking about genetic variants, it's common to hear about SNPs (pronounced "snips"), or single nucleotide polymorphisms. These are the most common type of genetic variation. They are single substitutions of one nucleotide (adenine, cytosine, guanine, thymine or A, C, G, T) on a piece of DNA. For example: a SNP might replace thymine with cytosine, or the other way around. Most SNPs have absolutely no effect on one's health. In fact, we each have between 4 and 5 million SNPs in our genome, which make us unique, to say the least. When you take a DNA test like 23andMe or Ancestry, this is how your lineage is being traced. You are the sum of the SNP variants that you inherited from your mother and father. The contributions—the copies—from your parents are known as alleles. Similarly, you will have mutations that you pass along to your children. Fortunately, most SNPs are harmless; they don't affect the areas of the genes that create important proteins.

The study of SNPs is helping scientists understand how you might respond to a particular medication, an environmental toxin, or a specific food. These very common genetic variations can alert us to an increased risk for developing a certain disease. Profiling these SNPs can also shed light on your skin beauty, whether you are at increased risk for wrinkling, pigmenting, glycating, or losing antioxidant ability; and with this information in hand, can help you choose specific nutrients that can help slow down these signs of aging.

Notice, in my discussion about genes, I often use words like risk, probability, and susceptibility. This is because genes are predictive, they are not diagnostic. Just because you have a specific gene, it does not necessarily mean that the gene will be expressed. By "expressed," I mean that the gene ultimately turns on or off a protein that affects key cellular reactions. Genes are turned on or off by our environment—the food we eat, the air we breathe, the toxins that into which we come in contact with. This influence is what is known as epigenetics. The genes themselves are not changed, just their expression. Many clinicians who study this area will often remark that "Genes load the gun, but environment pulls the trigger." While I'm not a big fan of gun or military analogies, this does bring home the critical point.

A classic example of epigenetic effects is the APOE4 gene which has been shown to increase the risk for dementia.[78] About 25% of people carry one copy of APOE4. About 2 to 3 percent of people have two copies of APOE4. Studies show that up to 60 percent of the two-copy group will develop Alzheimer's dementia by age 85, compared with 10 to 15 percent of the general population. If we flip the statistics around, 40% of people with the highest risk profile don't go on and get dementia. The APOE4 gene is there, but it is not being expressed in a way that causes harm. For this 40%, their lifestyle and diet has most likely protected them.

The Two-Way Street of Nutrition and Genes

Those of us who want radiant skin need to appreciate the two-way interaction of genes and foods, the science of which is known as nutritional genomics. This is shown in the diagram on the next page.

Nutrigenetics examines how your genes impact your response to nutrients and the bioactive compounds in food. Nutrigenetic examples include genes (in parenthesis) that can shed light on the following:

- Alcohol tolerance (ALDH2)
- Lactose intolerance (MCM6)
- Vitamin A (BCM01)
- Vitamin D (GC)
- Sugar preference (GLUT2)
- Caffeine metabolism (CYP1A2)
- Weight regain (ADIPOQ)
- Vitamin B12 (FUT2)
- Folate levels (MTHFR)
- Taste perception (CD36)

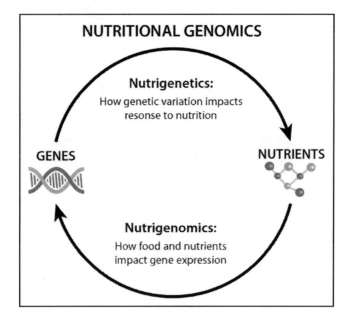

Genes can Help Clear up Nutritional Confusion

If you're like most people, when it comes to food recommendations, there is no shortage of confusion. Take coffee, for example. One study says it's good for you—loaded with antioxidants that promote health. The next study says it's going to shorten your life by leading to a heart attack or stroke. Which position is right? And what is best for you? The answer may lie in your genes, and in how, if you have inherited a certain profile, your response may differ from other people.

Ahmed El-Sohemy, PhD, is a professor of nutritional sciences at the University of Toronto. His lab was the first to explore the genetic link between genes and how the body handles caffeine. Caffeine is broken down by enzymes in the liver. A gene called CYP1A2 determines how well these enzymes work. If you have the fast-metabolizing variant, then your body can easily handle caffeine, and in this case, the substance provides health benefits. I often give great thanks to my parents for gifting me this genetic profile, as I'm sure I would never be able to complete writing a book without it. On the other hand, if you have the slow-metabolizing variant, and lack the ability to break down caffeine, it accumulates in your system and can be harmful. The graphs below show Dr. El-Sohemy's research. You'll note the inflection point around 1-2 cups a day, beyond which those with the slow-metabolizing variant should stop their consumption.

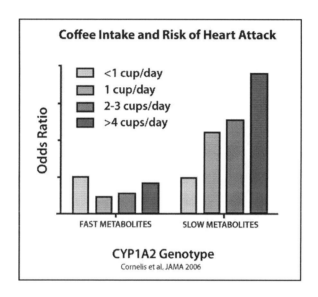

GENES FOR SKIN HEALTH & BEAUTY

Genetic tests differ in the number of genes they measure, the ones they report, and how the results are communicated. More than 77,000 genetic tests are currently in use.[79] The tests look for variants in a select number of genes. Increasingly, genetic testing is being done using whole genome sequencing, sometimes called exome sequencing. This analyzes the bulk of an individual's DNA to identify genetic variants. An example of a company that does whole genome sequencing is New Amsterdam Genomics (nagenomics.com).

Some panels of tests are offered exclusively to medical practitioners; however, increasingly companies are making varieties of gene panels directly available to consumers. The professionally-directed tests often include much more detailed analysis, such as better pinpointing the region of the gene that is affected. Physicians also will have your medical history, physical examination, and laboratory findings to factor into your nutrition plan. All of this can help the practitioner create more specific, personalized treatments.

Many of the direct-to-consumer genomic testing companies also offer their own supplement product lines. In many cases, the revenue from the supplements allows the company to offer their testing direct to you at lower prices. Some companies may also connect you with a dietitian, who may or may not be specifically trained in personalized nutrition.

There are trade-offs in determining which route to go. Getting your analysis done by a professional will usually be more expensive, but you'll get a more medically sound approach. Some of the consumer tests, and a few of the professional versions, will allow you to import your 23andMe data into their analysis, thus saving you some cost. At the conclusion of this chapter, I've listed a handful of the DTC companies and briefly described their offers.

Genes, Nutrition and Your Skin

Nutrition gene tests help you understand how your body responds to common foods and to make personalized recommendations for improving skin health. Several genetic variants are associated with loss of skin elasticity, diminished antioxidant capacity (reduced ability to neutralize free radical damage to the skin), wrinkle formation, and skin diseases. A nutritional genomics panel categorizes susceptibility as either typical risk or elevated risk for skin aging. If you have an elevated risk due to a specific gene variant, re-orienting your food, mineral, vitamin, and antioxidant selection may help you minimize the signs of skin aging and maintain a more youthful appearance. Of course, it's better to get a jumpstart when you're young. Decades of missing out on certain nutrients could potentially make you look much older than your chronological age.

For much of the content below, I am going to be drawing from the nutritional genomics report from the company Dr. El-Sohemy founded, Nutrigenomix (nutrigenomix.com). Nutrigenomix is the leading professionally oriented gene testing company, with over 10,000 skilled professionals available to access on their find-a-practitioner locator. In addition to offering a much larger panel tied to health habits and risks, Dr. El-Sohemy has created a specific test that looks at skin health and beauty-related SNPs. A few things to keep in mind as you read through the rest of this chapter:

- The names of genes are combinations of letters and numbers and are always capitalized.
- Genes "code" or "encode" for a protein or an enzyme. (Think: "have the potential to make" a protein or enzyme.) Genes also "express" a change. (Think: "cause to happen.")
- Remember, genes are predictive, and not diagnostic.
- The different configurations of genes you inherited are linked to different levels of risk for skin aging.
- Some genes accelerate biochemical reactions in the body. Other genes halt or slow these reactions.
- Because the major genetic drivers of skin aging are all accelerated by UVA/UVB exposure you'll want to be religious in your use of sunblock. I'll have more to say about this in PART III: What Topicals Should I Apply?

GO EASY ON YOUR BRAIN!

Unless you are a clinician, you'll most likely never repeat the names of the genes so often as to imprint them in your mind and let them roll easily off your tongue. Whenever you see the "alphabet soup" name of the gene in the text below, just replace it with "there is a gene that…" Think of this listing of genes as a reference guide that you can discuss with your clinician.

MAJOR GENETIC VARIANTS AFFECTING SKIN HEALTH

Collagen & Elastin Loss

A variant in the MMP1 (Matrix Metalloproteinase 1) gene affects the enzyme matrix metalloproteinase-1, which in turn, increases deterioration of the collagen and elastin fibers in skin. Collagen loss leads to wrinkles and furrows; elastin loss leads to skin laxity (sagging skin). Exposure to UV light only compounds the genetic variant's deleterious effect on the skin by accelerating the signs of aging.

If the genetic propensity for collagen and elastin degradation wasn't bad enough, we need to factor in the effects of glycation and advanced glycation endproducts (AGEs) discussed earlier. When collagen fibers are glycated, their structure changes; what was once a soft and supple texture, now becomes rigid and hard. This is most visible on areas with thin skin, such as the neck ("turkey neck"). Of course, unhealthy lifestyle factors—smoking, early-life sunburns, and excessive sun exposure—don't help.

Photoaging

The MC1R (Melanocortin 1 Receptor) gene has the unique task of giving us our skin, hair, and eye color. Variants make us different in our appearance. MC1R provides the instructions to make the protein melanocortin 1 receptor, which is involved in normal pigmentation. This gene controls melanin production within the melanocytes. The melanocytes synthesize 2 different types of melanin—pheomelanin and eumelanin. Individuals with the pheomelanin-dominant variant have blond or red hair, freckles, and fair or light-colored skin. Their skin is more likely to burn than tan when exposed to sunlight and, as such, have a high risk of UV skin damage. Individuals with the eumelanin-dominant variant typically have brown or black hair and darker skin tones; their skin tans easily and doesn't burn as much due to the eumelanin's protection against UV damage.

As you'd expect, fair-skinned people are much more likely to develop melanoma (skin cancer). Insufficient eumelanin makes them more vulnerable to damaging UV radiation, but this doesn't mean that darker-skinned people are completely protected against melanoma either. Additional variations in the MC1R gene, plus two other related genes (BRAF and CDKN2A), are likely to play a role in melanoma development even with no UV-induced skin damage. This is the reason it's possible to develop melanoma on the soles of the feet, which are hardly ever exposed to sunlight.

More bad news. Two common variants identified in the MC1R gene increase the risk for severe photoaging in women.[80] This is even the case when researchers account for other factors, like age, body mass index, skin phenotype, or menopausal status. That is to say, these two genetic variants have a lot of independent impact on skin aging. If you have the risk variants, it's more important that you do all the things we know to be good for the skin to limit the potential expression of these genes.

Facial Pigmented Spots

The variants in the IRF4 (Interferon Regulatory Factor 4) gene, as well as other genes relevant to skin color (MC1R, ASIP, and BNC2), contribute to pigmented spots (solar lentigines and seborrheic keratosis) on the face or neck which are associated with aging. Solar lentigines are the result of sun exposure and are commonly referred to as "dark spots." Seborrheic keratoses are waxy-looking, slightly-raised growths that can be colored light tan, brown, or black; they are non-cancerous, but can cause angst for people who find them unsightly. They are more prevalent in women. Research suggests that these variants influence the development of pigmented spots, not through the amount of melanin in the skin, but perhaps through the amount of cumulative UV damage.[81] Another hypothesis is that the skin is less effective at repairing itself from the damage caused by free radicals.

If you have blue eyes, brown hair and freckles, you most likely have the IRF4 variant.[82] So, if you don't have pigmented spots yet, you know what's potentially coming. Take care with your sun exposure and eat plenty of antioxidant-rich foods.

Oxidative Stress-Induced Premature Aging

The SOD2 (Superoxide Dismutase 2, mitochondrial) gene is important to the health of most cells in the body, including the skin. This gene codes for a key enzyme SOD that protects against oxidative stress, inflammatory proteins, and ionizing radiation. SOD2 is expressed in the mitochondria, and its function is to process superoxide, a toxic byproduct created by the mitochondria during the course of generating energy for the cell.

Superoxide (Think of it as a "super oxidant.") gets processed into less toxic components which are then expelled from the mitochondria. Essentially, SOD2 takes out the garbage generated by the mitochondria, so the mitochondria can continue to function without a buildup of garbage to impede or harm it. But, the SOD2 variant can result in either increased or decreased activity. Increased activity means the mitochondrial garbage is always taken out for recycling; decreased activity means the garbage accumulates and damages the mitochondria. It should also be noted that skin cells infected with *Propionibacterium acnes* produce superoxide radicals.

Oxidative Stress-Induced Premature Aging

The NQO1 (NAD(P)H Quinone Dehydrogenase 1) gene is similar to SOD2 with respect to the antioxidant capacity. It normally encodes for an enzyme (NQO1) which functions to rid the body of any partially oxidized quinone molecules that are otherwise highly reactive—in a bad way. And like SOD2, it scavenges for free radicals in the mitochondria and cell membrane to help protect the cells and tissues from oxidative damage. Individuals with the variant are more prone to damage and premature aging of the skin caused by free radicals. Ongoing exposure to sunlight, pollution, and cigarette smoking makes it worse.

Advanced Glycation Endproducts (AGE) Formation

The GLO1 (Glyoxalase 1) gene encodes for an enzyme (GLO1) that protects cells from advanced glycation endproducts (AGEs) and one specific AGE which is highly damaging—methylglyoxal. The GLO1 variant decreases GLO1 activity in the blood, resulting in more AGEs available to bind to collagen and elastin and cause skin cell damage which over time, leads to fine lines, wrinkles and sagging skin.

GENE	INDICATOR	RISK VARIANT PREVALENCE (ethnicity)*
GLO1	Advanced Glycation End Products	1 in 3 Europeans or Hispanics 1 in 2 East Asians or Africans
GLUT2	Sugar Preference	1 in 4 Europeans 1 in 3 Hispanics 3 in 4 Africans
IRF4	Facial Pigmented Spots	1 in 10 Africans 1 in 7 Hispanics 1 in 4 Europeans
MMP1	Loss of Elasticity	1 in 10 East Asians 1 in 6 Hispanics 1 in 4 Africans or Europeans
SOD2 & NQO1	Antioxidant Capacity	1 in 3 other ethnicities 2 in 3 East Asians

*Adapted from Nutrigenomix

Low GLO1 expression can be problematic for patients who have uncontrolled diabetes, chronic hyperglycemia (high blood sugar levels), or consume a lot of sweets and sugary beverages. Avoiding dietary sources of AGEs (sugar, BBQed meats, deep fried foods) is advised for anyone with this variant—and really everyone else—to prevent or reduce the amount of oxidation and inflammation throughout the body, not just the skin.

A related gene, GLUT2 (**Glu**cose **T**ransporter type 2) is expressed in the areas of the brain which influence our food preferences. This variant induces a personal preference for sweet foods and beverages, and individuals with the variant are more likely to overindulge. An excessive formation of AGEs can result as a consequence. Having both the GLO1 and GLUT2 variants makes it all that more important to watch your diet if you want to have great looking skin.

OTHER GENETIC VARIANTS AFFECTING SKIN HEALTH

Folate Deficiency

A variant in the MTHFR (*Methylenetetrahydrofolate Reductase*) gene impairs the body's ability to convert dietary folate to its active enzyme form—methylenetetrahydrofolate reductase. With this variant, individuals can become folate-deficient, especially if the amount of dietary folate is low. A minimum of 400 mcg/day of folate from food sources (lentils, edamame, asparagus, chickpeas, and cooked spinach) or supplements is necessary to offset the risk of deficiency.

A folate deficiency is typically associated with neural tube defects (i.e., spina bifida) in a developing fetus. Along with vitamins B6 and B12, low folate also corresponds to elevated homocysteine levels which has been implicated in numerous chronic health conditions. But what might be lesser known is folate's role in skin health, and specifically the genetic relationship to skin color.

One variant in the MTHFR gene has been proposed as contributing to the development of vitiligo, an autoimmune condition characterized by depigmented whitish skin patches.[83] Patients with vitiligo have elevated homocysteine levels, as do patients with plaque psoriasis. While not absolutely conclusive, research suggests that there is a relationship between the MTHFR variant and the severity of psoriasis.[84] If you or someone you know has either vitiligo or plaque psoriasis, testing should include an assessment of the MTHFR gene variants, as well as serum levels of cysteine.

High levels of oxidized cysteine in the blood cause white cells to send out inflammatory signals.[85] Your physician can check your cysteine levels and use these measurements to monitor how well antioxidants are working to reduce inflammation within your body. For those with skin conditions related to the MTHFR gene, supplementation with folate and vitamins B6 and B12 may be helpful.

I want to note that the body reacts differently to various stimuli (inputs) and of course, not everybody's body reacts the same. (Think: N of 1.) Mix in the gene variants, and it gets even more complicated.

Vitamin A Deficiency

Vitamin A (beta-carotene) is an antioxidant powerhouse that supports vision, teeth and bone growth, hormone production, and immune function, as well as skin health. Vitamin A deficiency (VAD) occurs infrequently in developed countries, and is common in vegans, which may seem odd because there are many vitamin A-rich foods for vegans to feast upon. But there is a reason. Animal sources such as eggs and fish already contain this active form, so it's more bioavailable from the start. The body is less efficient at breaking down plant sources, such as carrots and sweet potatoes, and converting the beta-carotene to the active form of vitamin A (retinoic acid). Therefore, vegans and perhaps some vegetarians tend to be low on vitamin A.

The likelihood that a vegan will have VAD is further increased if he or she has a variant in the BCO1 (Beta-Carotene Oxygenase 1) gene. Normally, the BCO1 gene produces an enzyme protein (BCMO1) which helps convert beta-carotene into retinoic acid. Obviously, VAD affects non-vegans who also carry this genetic variant. Without sufficient vitamin A in the body, the skin suffers from the lack of free-radical squelching antioxidants. For our vegan friends with the BCO1 variant, I suggest a lycopene supplement to satisfy your daily requirement.

Vitamin C Deficiency

The GSTT1 (Glutathione S-transferase theta-1) gene encodes for an enzyme that helps the body utilize vitamin C. The GSTT1 gene is present in either of two forms—insertion ("on") or deletion ("off"). The deletion form is essentially nonfunctional and decreases the body's ability to process dietary vitamin C. An individual with the deletion variant will have less vitamin C circulating in the blood compared to an individual with the insertion variant despite ingesting the same amount of vitamin C. Because vitamin C is an antioxidant powerhouse and supports collagen formation, the RDA for vitamin C would not be sufficient for someone with the deletion variant. So, get extra vitamin C from sweet red peppers, citrus fruits and juices, strawberries, pineapple, and Brussels sprouts. Because vitamin C can't be stored by the body, taking 1,000 mg a day of vitamin C will provide adequate protection for all.

Vitamin D Deficiency

The CYP2R1 (Cytochrome P450 2R1) gene encodes for the CYP2R1 enzyme which is expressed by the liver and secreted into the bloodstream. CYP2R1 is necessary to convert dietary vitamin D or vitamin D synthesized in the skin into calcifediol, the form which goes to the kidneys where it is transformed into the bioactive form of vitamin D_3 (calcitriol). Then, calcitriol helps the calcium from foods be absorbed in the gut and utilized in bone formation and muscle function. The CYP2R1 variant results in lower quantities of vitamin D_3 circulating in the blood, or vitamin D_3 inadequacy.

Another gene, the GC gene, also encodes for the vitamin D-binding protein which is expressed in the liver and secreted into the bloodstream. Once in the bloodstream this protein meets up with calcitriol. In an Uber-like fashion, the vitamin D-binding protein transports the calcitriol to the tissues where it assists in calcium absorption. The GC variant also reduces the amount of vitamin D_3 circulating in the blood. If you have either or both variants, consider getting more vitamin D from salmon, trout, halibut, milk, or fortified foods. It is difficult for people with a problematic SNP to maintain adequate levels of vitamin D through foods, so supplementation is important.

On a personal note, both my daughter and I have variants in our CYP2R1 and GC genes. Hence, even with an optimal diet, without supplementation we both maintain borderline deficient serum Vitamin D levels, measured in ng/mL, in the mid to high 20s. Vitamin D is a prohormone that is critical for immune health as well as bone formation. There are nearly 900 clinical studies highlighting the effect Vitamin D has on the immune system, with many showing that supplementation can help lessen the severity of COVID-19 infection. Knowing your level and optimizing it is quite important.

The Vitamin D Council, a nonprofit organization, recommends maintaining levels of 40–80 ng/ml (100–200 nmol/l) and states that anything over 100 ng/ml (250 nmol/l) may be harmful.[86] The rule of thumb that many clinicians use is 1,000-2,000 IUs/daily for each 10 ng/mL of deficiency. So, if your D_3 level is 30 and you want to get it to 60, taking 3,000 IU-6,000 IU daily should be adequate. NOTE: as a fat-soluble vitamin, Vitamin D takes longer to break down in the body, so you'll want to periodically measure your levels and keep supplementation reasonable.

Vitamin E Deficiency

The APOA5 gene participates in lipid (fat) metabolism and affects blood triglyceride levels. Triglycerides are the Uber/Lyft drivers for alpha-tocopherol, the most abundant form of bioactive vitamin E. Two copies of this variant result in lower blood concentrations of alpha-tocopherol than either one or no copies of the variant. Vitamin E is a powerful antioxidant, so if you have this variant, be sure to get the RDA from nuts, seeds, and healthy vegetable oils, and consider supplementing with vitamin E 400 mg (to be taken at mealtime). The vitamin E story is an unfolding one. I'll have more to say about it in the supplement chapter, where I'll discuss emerging research on the different types of vitamin E and their relationship to health and skin beauty.

Zinc Deficiency

The SLC30A3 (**Solute Carrier Family 30 Member 3**) gene encodes for one specific zinc transporter protein. (Think: Uber.) This affects zinc homeostasis in the blood. It also helps facilitate the release of stored zinc from cells for use in various metabolic processes. Two copies of the SLC30A3 variant are associated with lower blood levels of zinc, so be sure to consume at least the RDA (11 mg a day for men and 8 mg for women). Oysters, red meat, chicken, lobster, dairy products, and beans are excellent food sources. Even so, most people are deficient in zinc consumption, so additional supplementation with 30 mg/day can be helpful. Taking zinc as zinc carnosine can also help support the gastrointestinal tract.

For further information, please go to Appendix C.

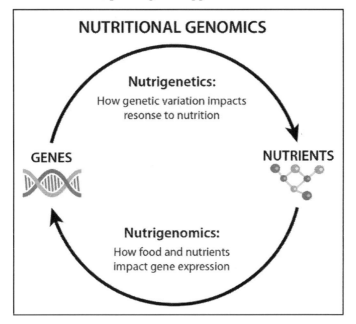

Nutrigenomics is the other side of the coin of the Nutritional Genomics story. This scientific discipline asks how nutrients act as dietary signals to impact gene expression. The best explanation of this emerging science is one offered by Jeffrey Bland, PhD, the founder of Functional Medicine. Speaking at the American Nutrition Association Summit in 2019, Dr. Bland declared:

> "We are a food-based culture. That is a shared common human experience. I've never met anyone who doesn't eat sometime, just like I've never met anyone who doesn't breathe sometime or I've never met someone who doesn't consume water sometime. There are shared common experiences that are essential for function…So, if we are a food-based culture, physiology is determined by the nutrients we consume…whose need for those nutrients is determined by the genotype of the individual. Therefore…food

represents the delivery system for nutrients that modulate an individual's phenotype, which is what we call nutrigenomics."

Simply put, within minutes to hours, the foods that you eat are either turning off or on key genes that regulate health or promote dysfunction.

The science behind foods specifically changing the genes for skin aging has lagged behind our clinical knowledge. We can draw some parallels from one of the most powerful studies showing the effect of lifestyle and nutrition in changing gene expression.[87] Dean Ornish, MD, and colleagues researched how a comprehensive lifestyle program could impact the genes that underlie prostate cancer. Dr. Ornish's patients strictly adhered to a low-fat diet with emphasis on mostly plant-based foods such as grains and beans, fruits, and vegetables. Participants (273 men with prostate cancer) in the Ornish Program agreed to walk a minimum of a half-hour per day, take stress management programs, do yoga or meditation, and attend a weekly support group. The combination of diet and lifestyle altered the activity of 500 genes, and the men showed significant improvements in their PSA levels, a marker for prostate cancer.

Just when you thought it couldn't get more complicated: There's another influential factor now included in emerging scientific concepts. The bacteria strains comprising the gut and skin microbiomes also have their own genes, which are similarly turned on or off depending on their environment. Their "environment" is the food that you eat. So rather than just say, *you are what you eat,* it may be more accurate to say *you are also what your gut bugs eat.* Your genes and those of the trillions of microbes in and on the human body together determine health, aging, vitality, and skin beauty.

The Emergence of Epigenetic Skin Tests

As skin cells differentiate, they undergo a set of metabolic changes that provide the biochemical and structural elements for an effective epidermal barrier. This process relies on gene expression, and it is highly affected by epigenetics. The most common biological process that drives this cellular differentiation is known as DNA methylation. It is the addition of methyl groups that change how the gene is expressed.

Over the last decade or so, researchers have been identifying and merging these methylation markers with artificial intelligence to predict how fast and how well a person is aging.[88] While every cell in the body has the same DNA, each cell has a different genetic identity. For example, because of epigenetics, heart tissue and skin tissue age at different rates.

According to Ryan Smith, VP of Business Development for TruDiagnostic (trudiagnostic.com), there are three artificial intelligence algorithms currently in use to predict aging. TruDiagnostic has been training one of them to specifically predict skin aging. The company anticipates having its skin aging epigenetic test available to clinicians toward the end of 2022. The test, which will involve a tape strip to collect the skin sample, will be able to evaluate parameters such as rate of wrinkling, pigmenting, and loss of volume.[89]

In this chapter, I've discussed a few of the many genetic variants that make each of us unique in terms of skin health. Of course, you need to be tested in order to know for certain whether you carry any of the specific variants. I've compiled a list of the top 6 nutrigenomic tests currently available to consumers. They are available at different price points ($99 - $399). When you get your results back, consider the output as the scientific rationale for making healthier food choices and supplementing intelligently.

Nutrigenomix – Provides testing both to physicians and direct to the public. Consumers can select a physician to work with, or order the test direct and the company will provide a nutritionist to go over the results. Do not underestimate the value of having a trained clinician explain your genetic report. **NutriGenomix.com**

Nutrition Genome – A cheek-swab test that analyzes 100 genes. The service includes recommendations for blood work, toxins and foods to avoid, and a comprehensive report that covers analysis of digestion, energy, hormones, detoxification, cognitive health, and longevity. A toxin sensitivity report highlights chemical sensitivities and drug metabolism insights. The company does not offer supplements or analysis of previous DNA tests. **NutritionGenome.com**

My Toolbox Genomics – The consumer alternative to Toolbox Genomics (sold to practitioners). Offers three tests via saliva: the DNA test, an epigenetics test, and a combination of the two. The epigenetic report delivers information on biological age, cognitive health and risk, and genetic expression over time. Also provides customers with unique meal plans and exercise recommendations. Does not sell supplements or have data import capability. **MyToolBoxGenomics.com**

DNAfit – Three levels of tests and reports from a cheek swab. Basic kit provides diet-related feedback on food, fat, and carbohydrate sensitivity, toxin generation speed, and nutrient deficiency insight. Second level kit also includes fitness markers and a stress and sleep report. The Premium kit is a comprehensive screening with over 350 reports including cancer risk and cognitive health risk. Optional fitness consultations including live video calls and a custom week-long meal plan. Allows for import of your existing DNA information. **DNAFit.com/us**

Rootine – Combines a DNA cheek swab with an at-home finger prick that tests for vitamin D, B6, B9 (folate), and B12 levels. Provides basic information on micronutrient processing, cardiovascular health, brain health, bone health, vitamin deficiencies, and food sensitivities. They sell a custom vitamin packet based on results. The company does not offer data import. **Rootine.co**

Genopalate – Genopalate is a diet-focused nutritional genomic testing service that specializes in meal-based and supplement-based recommendations. The report, based upon a cheek swab, provides macronutrient ranges, sensitivities to gluten, lactose, and alcohol, as well as food and supplement intake suggestions. Offer supplemental nutrition related products. Provide vitamins and ability to import existing data. **GenoPalate.com**

Chapter 6

MANAGING YOUR HORMONES FOR SKIN & HAIR BEAUTY

Hormones? If you're a woman, you're probably thinking UGH, and if you're a man with women in your life—or if you're concerned about hair loss or sexual performance—you too are probably thinking UGH. There's no doubt that this chapter has its Venus-Mars undertones, and although the first part of this chapter is primarily geared towards women, men also experience hormone-related skin issues. But, more importantly, men can glean a better understanding of what women experience in mid-life and beyond, while learning to be more empathetic towards the women in their lives. This is my goal for my fellow men.

Hormones definitely affect the skin. Just think back to high school, puberty, and facial acne. It was a rough time for many…something we'd rather forget. Fast forward to adulthood and pimples pop back up, but this time, other unpleasantness accompanies the acne, especially for women as they age—dry skin, hot flashes, night sweats, difficulty sleeping, fatigue, mood swings, vaginal wall thinning and dryness, low libido, weight gain, anxiety, and depression. Again, it's the change in hormones—primarily declining estrogen levels—that come with perimenopause and menopause.

Sub-Optimal Hormone Levels & Premature Skin Aging

Even if women can successfully hide the sexual symptoms, sleep disturbances, and mood issues, it's exceedingly difficult to hide the skin changes associated with hormone imbalance. With aging, both women and men tend to experience hormone-related jowling (the noticeably sagging skin below your chin or jawline). However, for women, it tends to occur more noticeably and more dramatically around the time of menopause. Premature ovarian insufficiency, or "early menopause" which occurs in the fourth decade, increases facial aging and deterioration of soft and hard tissues of the face and elsewhere in the body. The sex hormones (estrogen and testosterone) are exceedingly influential throughout the lifespan of both sexes, and for women, most evident at puberty, pregnancy, and menopause.

Let's examine the 5 hormones that exert the greatest effect on skin. These include estrogen, progesterone, testosterone, thyroid hormones, and cortisol.

- **Too Little Estrogen:** Declining estradiol (a form of estrogen) production by the ovaries is the main cause of dry skin (loss of hydration) and sagging skin (loss of elasticity). The normal function of the various estrogens is to stimulate the skin cells (fibroblasts) to produce collagen and elastin. In the perimenopausal years, estrogen slowly tapers off, and this is when the skin begins to lose firmness, appear less vibrant, and develop fine lines which evolve into wrinkles. Estrogen loss accelerates during menopause, with a cessation in the postmenopausal years or at the time of a complete hysterectomy. Estrogen replacement is an option that women should always discuss with their healthcare providers (preferably a hormone specialist) whether for skin improvement and/or symptom management. Options include oral supplementation, topicals, and implantable pellets. (Refer to hormone replacement options in box.)
- **Too Little Progesterone After Menopause:** Progesterone protects the endometrial lining and prevents abnormal uterine bleeding (i.e., the uterus is still intact). Progesterone plays a role in collagen production, so the tapering off after menopause contributes to a loss of elasticity and increase in fine lines and wrinkles.
- **Too Much/Not Enough Testosterone:** One of the normal functions of testosterone is to stimulate sebum (oil) production which provides natural protection to the skin. If the normal and delicate balance between testosterone and estrogen gets out of whack, the skin may become abnormally oily, leading to acne. An imbalance can occur if estrogen levels drop while testosterone levels remain normal or just below normal levels. This is what happens in menopause. An excess of testosterone occurs in patients with polycystic ovary syndrome (PCOS) in women of childbearing age; increased body and facial hair (hirsutism) and acne are signs of PCOS. Although not as commonly

> **PROS & CONS OF HORMONE REPLACEMENT THERAPY OPTIONS**
>
> **PILLS:** Upside: pills are convenient.
> Downside: requires a daily regimen. Increases the risk of blood clots.
>
> **LOTIONS:** Upside: direct absorption into the skin.
> Downside: unpleasant smell; hormone may be transferred to partner.
>
> **PATCHES:** Upside: odorless direct absorption into the skin
> Downside: skin irritation, and roller coaster hormone levels in blood.
>
> **PELLETS*:** Upside: convenient, effective and lasts 3-4 months
> Downside: Requires an incision, low risk of infection and extrusion (pellet pops out).
>
> *Note: Many physicians are now utilizing the Pellecome® device that guarantees correct pellet placement and decreases the likelihood of extrusion and infection.*

diagnosed in women, low testosterone levels can contribute to symptoms of lethargy, sleep disturbances, weight gain, decreased libido, vaginal dryness, and menstrual irregularities.

- **Too Little Thyroid**: Low levels of thyroid hormones can make the skin dry, brittle, and pale. Low thyroid levels are not necessarily a result of menopause and can affect both women and men.
- **Too Much Cortisol**: Surges of the "stress hormone" cortisol can increase sebum production, triggering acne, and/or trigger inflammation. Chronically elevated cortisol levels can make inflammatory skin conditions, such as eczema, rosacea, vitiligo, as well as acne, worse. A secondary consequence is that high cortisol can stimulate sugar and carbohydrate cravings which in turn, leads to glycated collagen as the skin loses flexibility and suppleness. There are also people who are "burned out" from chronic stress and no longer have much of a cortisol response. This too can trigger inflammation.

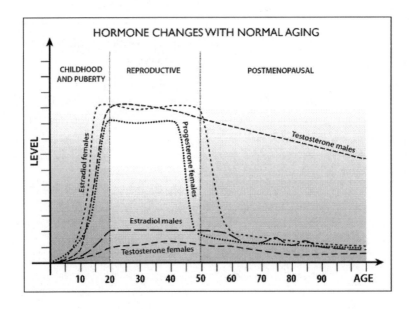

The body's ability to self-regulate its hormones is like a delicate, well-choreographed dance. Yet, when the dance gets off-kilter (i.e., perimenopause, menopause, postmenopause) a little, or a lot, hormone replacement therapy is always an option. Today, more women are opting for Bioidentical Hormone Replacement Therapy (BHRT). "Bioidentical" means that the hormones are chemically identical to the hormones produced in the body. "Natural" hormones are derived from plant or animal sources and are chemically processed to become "bioidentical."

Benefits of Hormone Replacement Therapy[90,91,92,93,94,95,96]
- Increased energy
- Improved sleep
- Relief of migraine or menstrual headache
- Relief from depression, decreased anxiety
- Increased muscle mass and bone density
- Decreased soft fatty tissue
- Increased coordination and physical performance
- Improved skin (increased collagen and elastin)
- Increased concentration and memory
- Improved overall physical health (blood pressure, lipids, glucose)
- Improved libido and sexual satisfaction
- No increased risk of strokes or blood clots

> **Women considering BHRT should have these tests performed by a doctor specializing in women's health:**
> - Free and total testosterone
> - Estradiol, FSH (follicle stimulating hormone)
> - Progesterone
> - DHEA (another sex hormone)
> - Thyroid Hormones: TSH, free T4, free T3
> - CBC (Hb & Hct)
> - SHBG (Sex Hormone Binding Globulin, optional)
> - Comprehensive Metabolic Panel, Lipid Panel, HbA1C
> - Mammogram
> - Pelvic Ultrasound
> - Pap smear
>
> **Men considering BHRT should also have these tests (in addition to some above):**
> - PSA
> - Homocysteine

Hormone Imbalance & Acne

Now, let's drill down a bit on hormone imbalance and acne in women. Because menopause tips the delicate balance between estrogen and testosterone, adult acne can be problematic for women in their fifties…particularly when they don't expect to have acne at that stage of life. As mentioned previously, during menopause, women have less estrogen which changes the ratio to favor testosterone, and kickstarts acne formation. Also, if a woman has her ovaries and develops polycystic ovarian syndrome (PCOS), she is prone to developing acne and hirsutism. For some, this is distressing enough to seek medical help.

Too much testosterone can also cause or aggravate rosacea. Furthermore, women who are genetically-prone to high testosterone levels and very oily skin not only experience more cystic acne and breakouts on the chest and back, they often find that skincare products designed for oily skin are harsh and irritate their skin—after all, thinning skin is another effect of menopause. It may feel like a lose-lose situation, but it doesn't have to be if you look at the bigger picture. Sure, there's genetic susceptibility and natural hormonal changes, but you can help offset these symptoms through following a healthy lifestyle, practicing good nutrition, limiting toxin exposure, and adopting other health promoting factors that influence your "radiance quotient," or RQ. Your so-called "bad" genes don't necessarily get turned on unless you continually live in such a way that turns them on (i.e., smoking, excessive UV exposure, poor diet, inactivity).

Nutritional Approaches to Hormone Balance

Whether or not you decide to go on hormones to improve your skin's appearance (It's a very personal decision.), you can always modify your nutrition to enhance hormonal balance. It's a good strategy at any life stage where hormones may be affecting the look and feel of your skin—whether you're a woman or a man.

ESTROGEN	
If LOW: use herbs & botanicals, such as black cohosh, maca, hops; or use a phytoestrogen such as flaxseed.	If HIGH: eat cruciferous vegetables, seaweed, foods containing turmeric; take a supplement with DIM (diindolylmethane, found in cruciferous vegetables).
TESTOSTERONE	
If HIGH: use Reishi mushrooms, licorice root, green tea, spearmint.	For BALANCE: eat more foods with omega-3 fatty acids; or foods rich in zinc (pumpkin or sesame seeds, green beans); take a zinc supplement.
THYROID HORMONE	
If LOW: eat seaweed (for its iodine); eat fish, eggs, and nuts which are rich in omega-3 fatty acids and selenium.	If HIGH: eat antioxidant-rich foods, cruciferous vegetables, vitamin D-rich foods (fish, mushrooms); use non-iodized salt, if any. Avoid red, processed, and fried meats; high-glycemic carbs; alcohol and caffeine; and iodized salt.
CORTISOL	
If HIGH: avoid or limit alcohol, caffeine, sugar, and highly processed foods; use adaptogens such as ashwagandha, astragalus, ginseng, and rhodiola.	If LOW: drink morning licorice tea, or take adrenal glandulars.

Adult acne is generally considered a hormonal condition and the hormonal diagnostic avenue should be evaluated first. There can also be some influence from vitamin and mineral deficiencies. Low levels of antioxidant vitamins (A, C, D, E) may be due to insufficient dietary intake, but can also be caused by problems with the body's ability to absorb and utilize the vitamins. Without these vitamins, oxidative stress compromises the skin's protective barrier and contributes to breakouts. Although rare, a deficiency in some of the B vitamins can contribute to acne or produce acne-like symptoms. A zinc deficiency can play a role in both acne and dermatitis. Common causes include diabetes, liver disease, sickle-cell anemia, chronic diarrhea, and zinc malabsorption. Research involving zinc supplementation alone or as an adjunctive treatment has shown to be particularly effective in decreasing the number of pimples caused by acne.[97]

Not only is magnesium critical for overall health, but it provides foundational support for the production and activity of hormones. Magnesium helps the body make estrogen, progesterone, testosterone, and thyroid hormone. At the same time, magnesium prevents excessive cortisol production and calms the nervous system, and it helps balance blood sugar levels by controlling insulin secretion and reducing sugar cravings. These features can be quite helpful when dealing with hormonal issues—perimenopause, PCOS, PMS, thyroid disorder, adrenal fatigue, or anxiety.

Don't Forget About the Gut Microbiome

The premise of *Feed Your Skin Right* is to leverage today's nutrition knowledge to enhance your skin's appearance. In the last decade or so, we've gained a plethora of information about the body's various microbiomes—even though we've only scratched the surface. If you had acne as a teenager and your dermatologist prescribed oral antibiotics, it's likely that your gut microbiome was affected—and not in a good way, especially if you took them long term. You may even suffer the consequences of an unbalanced microbiome or a leaky gut today, and although there's no way to undo misguided behaviors of the past, we can make positive changes going forward. The probiotic supplements I mentioned in Chapter 3: The Power of Plant-Based Eating for Skin Beauty offer a good option for addressing adult acne, along with an optimized diet, of course.

Hair Today Doesn't Have to be Gone Tomorrow

On occasion, I am called upon at conferences to moderate clinician panel discussions on the relationship between hormones, nutrients, and hair restoration. I always point out the irony that I—the follicular-challenged doctor—get to guide the discussion, because, as my daughter is always pointing out, "This didn't work so well for you, Dad." The reality is that we know so much more about hair loss and hair restoration than we did when I experienced my fallout. Even though fortunately for me, the shaven head is all the rage.

The most common form of hair loss is known as androgenetic or androgenic alopecia, but more commonly known as male and female pattern loss. In men, hair loss occurs in a well-defined pattern, beginning above both temples. Over time, the hairline recedes to form a characteristic "M" shape. Hair also thins out at the crown. This may progress to partial or complete baldness.

The pattern of hair loss in women differs from male-pattern baldness. In women, the hair becomes thinner all over the head. The hairline remains intact. Androgenetic alopecia in women rarely leads to total baldness.

According to Terrence Keaney, MD, (skindc.com) a dermatologist, who specializes in hair restoration, "Hair loss is a misnomer. In fact, androgenetic alopecia patients aren't really losing their hair. Their hair is progressively miniaturizing. So, I like to say my patients are losing volume. The hair is occupying less space on their scalp, which results in more visible scalping exposed over time."

Hair Loss in Men

Dr. Keaney notes that, "Androgenetic alopecia is quite prevalent, especially in men where it coincides with their decade of life, affecting 20% of 20-year-olds, and 50% of 50-year-olds."

Most men have ample warning about their risk for male pattern balding. They need only look at how their fathers, siblings, and other relatives have fared. The goal is to maintain volume and stave off the thinning. The primary way this is done is through blocking the hormone dihydrotestosterone (DHT). This can be done either pharmaceutically, or nutritionally. You'll find my recommendations for hair growth supplements for both men and women at the end of this chapter.

The pharmaceutical options for men are somewhat limited. They include prescriptions for oral finasteride (Propecia®), which often has sexual side effects, as well as over the counter topical preparations of Minoxidil either as a lotion, shampoo, foam or spray.

Another option—to be discussed with your physician—is the application of compounded topic preparations. Sahar Swidan, PharmD, is a recognized expert in creating customized hair growth formulations. Speaking to the benefits of compounded topicals, she notes that, "Every drug has a single mechanism of action. The beauty of compounding is our ability to combine a number of substances, which together create synergy. We can combine pharmaceutical agents such as Minoxidil, retinoic acid, tretinoin, very low doses of finasteride, progesterone, or bimatoprost (the drug in the pharmaceutical lash-growing topical), along with nutritional components such as biotin which contributes to healthy hair, and niacinamide for greater blood flow. We can then formulate this personalized blend as a lotion, a foam, a gel, or a cream." If compounding seems interesting to you, you can learn more and encourage your physician to contact Dr. Swidan at sahar.world.

Needles and Hair Regrowth

Many men (and women as well) will turn to injections of platelet rich plasma (PRP). In this procedure, done by licensed healthcare practitioners, blood is collected via a venipuncture and then spun down in the tube. The layer that contains the growth factors from the platelets is withdrawn and injected into the scalp. Most doctors will recommend monthly injections for three months, followed by maintenance injections spaced 3-6 months apart.

The results for PRP are somewhat variable, depending in part on the volume and quality of the concentrate that is obtained. For men and women who have not had acceptable results with PRP, the difference may lie in the quality of the collection. One review examined 12 studies encompassing 295 patients treated with PRP and found that, "Hair count and thickness were visibly improved after 6 months of PRP treatment; approximately 40.6% of study participants reached at least a moderate level of improvement."[98]

Another treatment in the minimally-invasive category involves the use of micro-needling combined with the application of a hair regeneration-type serum. The serum, containing stem cell growth factors and cytokines, penetrates the scalp through the small channels created by the device. This is the basis for AnteAGE MD® hair treatment. The serum comes packaged with a micro-needling stamp which penetrates the scalp down to 0.25mm. Medical offices can use a deeper device than is available for home use. A number of dermatologists whom I respect are using this system in their practices with reportedly good results.

Female Hair Loss

While female pattern baldness is less common, many women are more attuned to the loss of their hair, either at times of great stress, or during the varying stages of menopause. They may first notice that their scalp part is becoming wider, or that they are seeing more hair on their brush or in the shower, or that their ponytail is thinning. Reena Jogi, MD, a double board-certified dermatologist and hair restoration specialist in Houston, TX notes that she is seeing an uptick in younger patients coming in to see her. She attributes this partially to awareness that there are more treatment options; even so, is surprised by how young some women are when they first experience hair loss.

Unlike men who have a predictable, familial pattern, Dr. Jogi points to the need to do a more extensive workup for women including a medical and medication history. She looks for drugs that can contribute to hair loss such as antidepressants and some blood pressure medications. She also checks thyroid levels, serum iron in young women, and zinc and B12 levels. Pharmaceutical options in women includes spironolactone which blocks androgens, and while the medication has few side effects, according to Dr. Jogi, "some women are averse to taking a medication." She also notes that the application of low-level laser therapy can aid in hair regrowth.

Healthy Hair from the Inside Out

Hair growth nutraceutical formulations are available both from medical professionals, and also sold directly to consumers. The formulations include a variety of active botanicals. The most common active ingredient in men's formulations is saw palmetto, which serves to block the hormone DHT, although there are other herbal DHT blockers. (Refer to the list on page 122.) DHT contributes to the hair follicles miniaturizing in men. Women who experience excess growth of facial hair, pubic hair, and acne around the time of menopause can also benefit from a natural DHT blocker. Women's formulations will often have ashwagandha, an adaptogen that helps reduce the cortisol stress response. Other ingredients may include antioxidants, probiotics, vitamins, and minerals.

Professional hair regrowth products with natural ingredients have been formulated and studied by dermatologists who carefully monitor and measure hair growth. These formulations are standardized, and there is rigorous attention to quality. Professionally developed formulations are further distinguished from some of the direct-to-consumer supplements by the clinical studies that support them, as well as the absence of pharmaceutical agents. The four most highly regarded professional hair regrowth formulations include:

- **Nutrafol®** (nutrafol.com): Their line of supplements is carried by more than 1500 doctors and dermatologists. The product is also available direct to consumers. Nutrafol sells patented supplements that have extensive clinical research behind them. The unique "secret sauce" is the Synergen Complex®, a standardized formula with patented stress adaptogens, DHT inhibitors and super antioxidants. For women, Nutrafol offers formulas depending on the stage of life when changing hormone levels are most influential— postpartum and perimenopause/postmenopause—as well as general hair support when stress and poor nutrition play a role in hair loss. Randomized, double-blinded clinical studies have shown improvement in the number and thickness of hairs.[99] Nutrafol for men targets hormonal imbalance, stress, and poor nutrition. (It doesn't compromise sexual function either.) The company has just introduced a growth activator serum with ashwagandha exosomes.

- **Viviscal™** (retail version) and **Viviscal™ Pro** (professional version) have solid clinical support backing their product, including 10 published clinical studies that have shown improvements in the number of hairs, increased hair thickening and decreased shedding.

- **Votesse™** (eclipsemedglobal.com/eclipse-votesse) is a proprietary supplement available only through medical professionals; it complements low-level laser therapy and other in-office hair re-growth procedures. In addition to the proprietary oral nutraceutical, the company features a topical foam.

- **Heilus No.1 Emerge-K** (heilus.com) is an oral supplement that provides digestible, functional keratin and cysteine. These ingredients have been shown to active skin cells to increase the body's production of collagen Types IV and VII, which are also critical for nail strength.

> **NATURAL DHT BLOCKERS**
> - Saw palmetto
> - Pumpkin seed oil
> - Pygeum
> - Fenugreek
> - Tea tree oil (topical)
> - Caffeine (topical)
> - Stinging nettle
> - Lycopene
> - Green tea
> - Soy
> - Lavender oil (topical)

There are other nutraceutical ingredients such as collagen and silicon that can contribute to both healthy hair and nails. We'll discuss these in PART II: What Supplements Should I Take?

Hormones: It's all a Matter of Balance

The major message I hope I've conveyed in this chapter is two-fold. First, hormones have an enormous impact on skin health and follicular abundance—even if ideas about "beauty" are mere reflections of our personal perceptions. Second, there are tangible, medically-supported options if you want to improve your appearance and in turn, your quality of life. My advice is to check with your primary care physician first and request a referral to an anti-aging or integrative practitioner who specializes in hormone replacement. Alternatively, you can use the Find a Practitioner link on the Pellecome.com site to find a qualified physician near you. In the meantime, utilize good nutrition and lifestyle habits. If you choose to feed your skin right, the hormone replacement aspect will simply enhance it.

Chapter 7

LIFESTYLE, VIBRANCY AND THE INNER GLOW

One of the great functional medicine physicians, David B. Wright, MD, from Premier Prevention in Memphis, TN, makes a profound statement to his patients:

"I can't out-prescribe your lifestyle."

I often find myself reflecting on this when people want the quick fix: the pill for instant weight loss, the prescription for anxiety, or medications for type 2 diabetes. Modifying lifestyle—through nutrition, stress management, physical fitness, and sound sleep habits—is so much more powerful than any pill for a chronic disease. For patients who choose to maintain unhealthy habits, there are no pills that will undo the powerful deleterious effects of how they live.

If I were to ask you to list the traits of the healthiest people you know, what adjectives would you use? Having asked this of tens of thousands of people over the years, the descriptor that is on everyone's list is *energy*: having enough of it to exceed the demands of life and work, being able to focus it, and turn it off when it's time to relax. No matter what you do for your skin, if you don't have energy, you won't radiate inner beauty.

This is where the mitochondria come in.

In the previous chapter, I briefly talked about the mitochondria and how an individual's genetic variants (SOD2 and NQO1) can influence mitochondrial efficiency and play a role in how well (or poorly) the skin ages. I didn't really get into the mitochondria themselves, but now's the time to drill down.

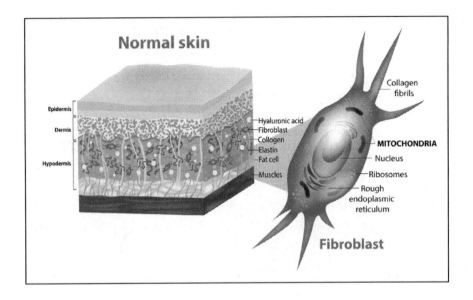

Maxing Out Your Mitochondria

Most of the body's cells contain mitochondria. These organelles (small organs) are responsible for the process known as cell respiration, or energy production. Mitochondria convert sugar and oxygen to carbon dioxide, water and fuel (energy called ATP) for the body to function. In fact, the mitochondria are referred to as the "powerhouses" of the cells. A skin beauty program both protects the mitochondria, and also enhances them.

When we talk about skin cells and photoaging, damaged mitochondria are involved in wrinkle formation, uneven pigmentation, hair loss, hair greying, and decreased wound healing.[100] They can become damaged as a result of oxidative stress related to normal aging, but also as a consequence of chronic inflammation and DNA damage related to smoking, UV radiation and pollution exposure.[101] Photoaging occurs when damaging UVA and IRA (near infrared) light penetrates into the dermis, causing a cascade of mitochondrial DNA damage and low-grade inflammation which only worsens with chronic UV exposure.

Mitochondrial Enhancement

As the mitochondria age (because you age), they slowly begin to release free radicals, or reactive oxygen species (ROS), which can then harm your skin (and other) cells. We call this "mitochondrial dysfunction" and it's one of the root causes of aging. Premature or accelerated mitochondrial dysfunction within the skin cells makes you look older because, in essence, your skin cells are getting older quicker.

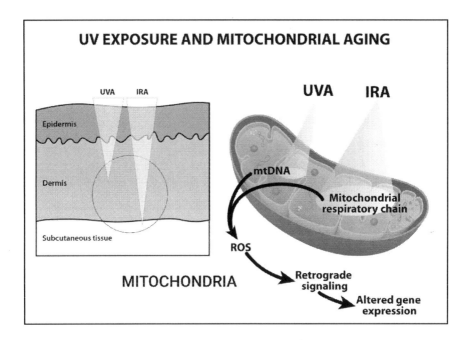

There are a number of well recognized supplements that can support mitochondrial health.[102] These include:

- **Alpha-lipoic acid** (ALA) is an antioxidant made naturally by the body and also found in food; it helps to break down carbohydrates for energy. In addition to helping with aging skin, it is also used for obesity, diabetes, and high cholesterol. Normal dosage is 600 mg, once or twice a day with meals.

- **Amino acids**: Arginine is used in the biosynthesis of proteins. It is essential for the body in order to synthesize nitric oxide, which maintains blood vessel health and aids in exercise and muscle performance. Citrulline is another amino acid that can help with muscle weakness. I recommend a powdered amino acid mixture called aminoLIFE™ (amino-life.com) which has been shown to support muscle growth.

- **B vitamins** including niacin, thiamin, riboflavin, and folic acid. A basic daily multivitamin or B-complex supplement with several times the recommended daily allowance is usually sufficient to maintain vitamin B levels.

- **Carnitine** is involved in metabolism where it transports fatty acids into the mitochondria to be used for fuel. Most people get adequate amounts from the diet.

- **Coenzyme-Q10** is a powerful antioxidant that protects cells from damage and plays a key role in metabolism. It is depleted in the body by statin drugs used to lower cholesterol. A typical daily dose is 100-200 mg/day. One supplement, MitoQ® combines Coenzyme-Q10 with a positive charge that allows for improved absorption into the mitochondrial membrane.

- **Vitamins C, E, & K** serve as important co-factors in energy reactions.

- **Magnesium** is also critical for mitochondrial function. I'll have much more to say about this key mineral in PART II: What Supplements Should I Take?

- **NAD+ (nicotinamide adenine dinucleotide)** is a critical coenzyme that is involved in hundreds of metabolic processes including repairing and protecting DNA, extracting energy from foods, preserving chromosome integrity, and maintaining mitochondria.

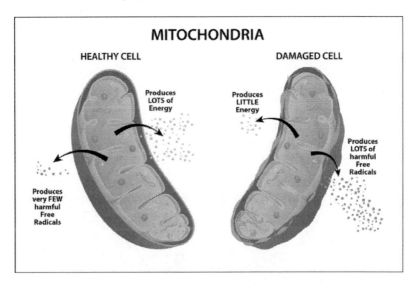

Exercise to the Rescue

Aside from a skin-healthy diet, not smoking, staying out of the sun, etc., exercise is great for taking care of your mitochondria—as long as you protect your skin when exercising outdoors. Exercise benefits the existing mitochondria by helping to stave off the otherwise "normal" loss in ability to produce ATP.

Exercise is good for your heart, lungs, and overall health, but it's also important for skin health. And the first reason is simple—blood flow. Exercise increases blood flow throughout the body which means oxygen and essential nutrients from a healthy diet are delivered to all cells and cellular waste products are removed. It's a win-win for your skin cells as well as just about every other cell in the body.

Some groundbreaking research in 2015 in both mice and humans showed favorable results at the mitochondrial level. Three months of endurance exercise (cycling) in otherwise sedentary elderly adults improved skin structure and increased mitochondria in the skin tissue.[103] The supposition is that regular exercise—longer than just 3 months—will elicit even better results and attenuate the progression of skin aging.

In addition to mitochondrial health, the age-related accumulation of advanced glycation endproducts (AGEs) is of interest to researchers trying to ascertain the benefits of regular exercise on skin. A 2014 study found that life-long endurance running helps counteract the progressive build-up of AGEs in connective tissue (Think: collagen in skin.) compared to sedentary individuals.[104] A 2019 study confirmed a modest decrease in glycation in long distance runners (of at least 10 years) who trained at least twice a week. Taken together, these studies suggest that it's never too late to begin an exercise regimen to promote skin health. Although, it's certainly better to incorporate regular physical activity from an early age and make a lifetime commitment.

Exercise, and weight-bearing exercise in particular, is important to maintain bone density as we get older. I'm not just talking about osteopenia and osteoporosis here, but facial bone retraction ("shrinkage"). Sagginess and droopiness results from some bone shrinkage and shifting in the face. Of course, this can be accentuated by rapid or significant weight loss; facial tone becomes increasingly lax due to the loss of overlying soft tissue (fat and muscle). Even in the absence of weight fluctuations, the normal shifting of facial bones can have an effect on the position of soft tissue.[105] This process occurs throughout adulthood, with women experiencing more dramatic changes than men.

Exercise and Bone Health

Bone tissue throughout the body is continually being affected by two types of cells: osteoblasts which build bone tissue and osteoclasts that break it down. During youth, these two processes are well-matched, at times favoring osteoblast activity. Good skeletal structural support typifies this stage in life. By midlife, osteoclast activity begins outpacing the osteoblast activity, and as normal aging progresses, bone retraction accelerates. Although loss of soft tissue occurs almost universally, researchers have found that it is the bone loss in specific areas of the facial skeleton that contribute most to the aged appearance.[106] Walking, jogging, lifting weights, and other resistance exercise promotes osteoblast activity, which fortifies the skeleton in general and may fight gravitational effects on the face—or at least slow it down a bit.[107]

Exercise also has a positive impact on the gut microbiome by encouraging greater microbial biodiversity.[108] So, not only does it help the gut to function normally, exercise helps ensure the appropriate communication along the gut-brain-skin axis. Since the "good" gut bacteria help keep inflammation in check, then exercise could be utilized as a "treatment" for inflammatory-related skin conditions. The only word of caution concerns intense, prolonged exercise, such as marathons, triathlons, and similar activities, which has been shown to increase intestinal permeability ("leaky gut").[109]

There's more good news about the stress-relieving effect of exercise on certain skin conditions. Whether structured or recreational or just simple movement, physical activity helps decrease mental and emotional stress, which already tend to trigger or exacerbate inflammatory skin conditions. One acne hypothesis is that an increase in the stress hormone levels causes the skin's sebaceous glands to produce more oil. Stress can also worsen eczema in some people, and interestingly, research shows a link between the stress experienced by pregnant or postpartum women and the risk that their child develops eczema.[110] In this case, exercise as a stress reduction technique is good for your *child's* skin.

Again, I remind you that the brain and skin are inextricably linked via their bidirectional connection to each other and to the gut. We can debate—as has been done by scientists—whether mental stress causes skin problems or whether skin problems cause mental stress. It's some of both, and it characterizes the fascinating field of psychodermatology. But, in any case, exercise does appear to help ease stress.

> ### THE CALMING POWER OF HRV TRAINING
> On par with exercise's stress-relieving benefits are mindfulness practices, such as reflection and gratitude. When paired with deep rhythmic breathing, these practices calm the mind and increase heart rate variability (HRV). HRV is a measurement of the time interval between heartbeats. A high HRV (greater variability between each heart beat) is associated with greater cardiovascular fitness, a lower risk of death, and more resilience to stress. A low HRV (a more regular interval between each heartbeat) is associated with not simply increased risk of cardiovascular disease and heart attack, but also worsening anxiety, depression, or emotional strain. Consciously manipulating HRV is the rationale behind HeartMath®—self-regulating out of a stressful state into an emotionally calm and stable state.[111] Calming the mind helps regulate and improve the "brain" part of the gut-brain-skin axis.

A Good Night's Sleep is Mitochondria Regeneration Time

We're all a little cranky if we don't get enough sleep, and others around us know it. But the mitochondria suffer in silence when you don't get those ZZZs. The body's housekeeping (autophagy) occurs while you sleep, so falling asleep and staying asleep long enough for this to happen is critical. During sleep, hormones are released which promote the repair and growth of the cells comprising various tissues and organs in the body, including the skin. If you exercised intensely the previous day, sleep is even more important—to the damaged muscle cells in particular; they repair and regenerate so you can work out the following day. Studies show that a lack of sleep, sleep inefficiency, and/or abnormal sleep patterns (i.e., sleep apnea) can negatively affect the mitochondrial DNA. Poor sleep causes mitochondrial stress, which can, in turn, negatively affect health and longevity.[112]

We know that insufficient sleep causes the mitochondria to get a little cranky, but science is now beginning to think that the relationship also works in the opposite direction—cranky mitochondria interfere with sleep.

Animal studies suggest that mitochondria may play a role in the body's sleep-wake cycle, or circadian rhythm.[113] The circadian rhythm appears to have influence over the abundance (or lack) of mitochondria. More research is necessary to determine the exact mechanisms, but getting sufficient, good quality sleep should be one of the key components of a wellness-oriented lifestyle. Crankiness leads to frowns and scowls, which don't do anyone's appearance any favors.

> **General Guidelines for Adults* from the**
> *2nd Edition of Physical Activity Guidelines for Americans*
>
> - Adults should move more and sit less throughout the day. Some physical activity is better than none. Adults who sit less and do any amount of moderate-to-vigorous physical activity gain some health benefits.
>
> - For substantial health benefits, adults should do at least 150 minutes (2 hours and 30 minutes) to 300 minutes (5 hours) a week of moderate-intensity, or 75 minutes (1 hour and 15 minutes) to 150 minutes (2 hours and 30 minutes) a week of vigorous-intensity aerobic physical activity, or an equivalent combination of moderate- and vigorous-intensity aerobic activity. Preferably, aerobic activity should be spread throughout the week.
>
> - Additional health benefits are gained by engaging in physical activity beyond the equivalent of 300 minutes (5 hours) of moderate-intensity physical activity a week.
>
> - Adults should also do muscle-strengthening activities of moderate or greater intensity and that involve all major muscle groups on 2 or more days a week, as these activities provide additional health benefits.
>
> * For other age groups and those with chronic health conditions, view the complete report at: https://health.gov/our-work/physical-activity/current-guidelines

Exercise Guidelines for Good Health & Great Skins

The latter half of the 20th century and first part of the 21st century have seen a major shift towards a sitting culture. Our sedentary lifestyle is reflective of sitting as we go to and from work (in our cars), sitting at work (at our desks), and sitting at home (on our couches) in the evening as we recuperate from an entire day of…sitting. In 2018, the US Department of Health and Human Services published physical activity guidelines for people to help improve health and avoid chronic disease. If you're not already engaged in regular physical activity, I encourage you to first check with your primary care physician for approval. Then find a few activities that you enjoying doing and incorporate them into the guidelines on the previous page.[114]

In some patients with rosacea, psoriasis, or acne, exercise can cause flare-ups, so it's advisable to consult with your dermatologist. This is often caused by an increase in body temperature and/or oxidative stress. The overall benefits of regular exercise on the entire body are so tremendous that it's better to manage the unpleasant symptoms than forgo exercise entirely. Here are some general guidelines to protect your skin:

Rosacea[115]

- Consider the outdoor climate. When the weather is warm or hot, limit your outdoor exercise to the early morning or evening; avoid peak heat times. Aim for shaded walking or cycling trails and avoid hot asphalt. Wear lightweight, breathable clothing, a hat, and sunscreen.
- Adjust the indoor climate. Maintain a comfortable, well-ventilated room for indoor exercise.
- Choose low-impact activities. A low-impact workout is less likely to cause overheating, especially when done in a cool and comfortable indoor or outdoor climate.
- Combat the flushing. Place a damp, cool towel around your neck as soon as you feel your body heating up. Alternatively, spray mist your face with cold water, or chew/suck some crushed ice. Water aerobics and swimming are good choices.
- Divide up your workout. Instead of 45 minutes of continuous exercise do 2 or shorter segments to avoid overheating.

Eczema & Psoriasis[116]

- Sun in moderation. Sunlight can improve psoriasis but mild sunburn can aggravate it. Exercise in non-peak sunlight times (peak sunlight is usually 10am to 4pm, depending on where you live). Wear sun-reflecting clothing and apply a sunblock to exposed areas.
- Exercise in comfort. A cool or airconditioned environment helps prevent excessive perspiration. If you're prone to sweating, apply a moisturizer to counterbalance the salt in perspiration that can irritate the skin.
- Get loose. Tight-fitting clothing can irritate skin affected by psoriasis. Wear clothes made of cotton or moisture-wicking materials that fit loosely. Working out at home may allow you to wear less-restrictive clothing (or none at all).
- Go for a swim. Swimming and water aerobics are great if done in a salt-water pool; the salt helps slough off dead skin. Chlorine-treated pools should be avoided because chlorine can irritate your skin. If you do swim in a chlorinated pool, shower immediately afterwards and apply moisturizer.

Acne[117]

- Dab, don't rub. If you sweat during exercise, use a towel to gently dab your moist skin. Avoid rubbing as it may cause further irritation.
- Keep skin drier. Minimize perspiration during a workout with moisture-wicking clothing and exercise in a cool environment if possible. Shower immediately afterwards.
- Coordinate exercise with a topical anti-acne regimen. Because experts recommend washing acne-prone skin no more than twice daily, time your exercise with your cleansing schedule. Shower or wash your face after exercise—either in the morning or evening; then apply prescribed acne medications. A number of companies make cleansers with salicylic acid which helps shed the dead skin that blocks pores. These include iS Clinical® Cleansing Complex (isclinical.com), Murad® Clarifying Cleanser (murad.com), and SkinCeuticals® LHA Cleanser (skinceuticals.com).
- Low-intensity controls cortisol. Reducing inflammation by minimizing cortisol levels in the body can prevent acne in some people. If high intensity exercise is your trigger, stay with a low-intensity workout.

- Begin slowly and ramp up gradually. Intense workouts aren't necessarily off-limits but sporadic, intense exercise is likely to worsen acne. If you like an intense workout, start at low-to-moderate intensity and work your way up while being consistent.

TIPS TO OVERCOME A SEDENTARY WORKDAY

1. If your office building has an elevator, use the stairs instead. Park closer to the back of the parking and walk.
2. If you sit for extended periods, stand up and stretch every 30 minutes. Better yet, walk around your floor if possible.
3. Clench and release your buttock muscles 10 times, followed by 10 shoulder rolls to the back then to the front per hour.
4. Use an adjustable standing or treadmill desk.
5. Take a 10-to-15-minute brisk walk during your lunch break.

Before we close out PART I: What Should I Eat? and move on to supplement recommendations, I'd like to once more reinforce the power of eating nutrient-rich foods. As the name implies, supplements do just that—they *supplement* the diet. And there's not much sense in supplementing the SAD, if that's your current eating style. No amount of supplemental vitamins can make the SAD healthy.

Instead, choose a diet that is slanted towards plant-based foods—ones that are mostly whole, minimally processed, and organically or backyard grown. If you feed your skin right, it (and your entire body) will function more optimally and protect you from the outside environment. You'll have that natural glow which exudes health, well-being, and aesthetic attractiveness.

Part Two: What Supplements Should I Take?

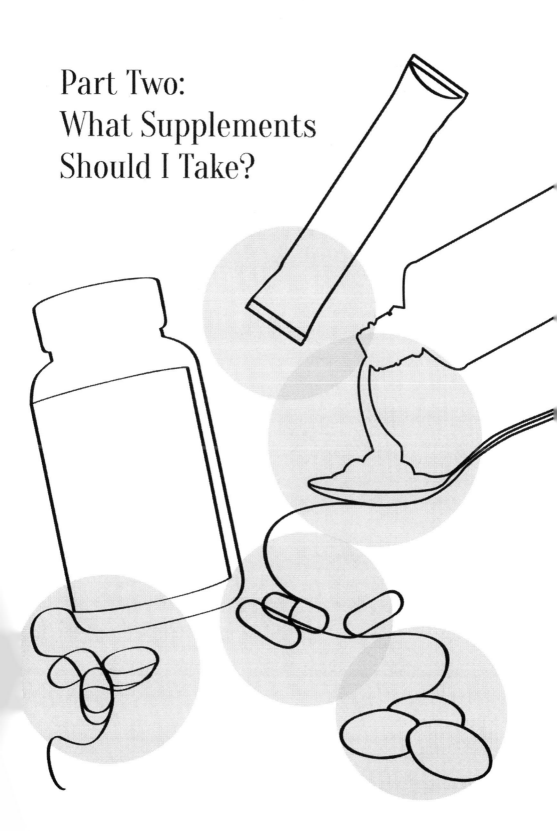

*"Beauty is about enhancing what you have.
Let yourself shine through."*

Janelle Monáe

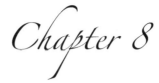

SETTING THE RECORD STRAIGHT ON SUPPLEMENTS

I pride myself on generally being a calm, level-headed guy. My wife will often refer to me as being "Buddhistic," meaning, like the Buddha, I tend to roll with life's punches. I do recall one time when I was really pissed off. It involved:

1. A well-known cardiologist and best-selling author at a prestigious medical establishment;
2. A talk he was giving for which I was in the audience; and
3. A statement he made in a rather blanket fashion: "Americans don't need to take supplements, they just excrete them in the urine. Americans have the most expensive urine in the world."

I bit my tongue and to this day, regret that I didn't challenge this physician. As a partial excuse, we were in his town. Clearly, he was overlooking a few key points in his synthesis. Namely, he excluded from his generalization some, if not all, of the following:

- People who live in cold climates in the winter. Check the vegetable aisle in January, February, and March and you'll find very little produce that is a deep shade of green. Grown in nutrient-depleted soil, picked early, trucked in, subject to oxidation, fiber still intact while other bioactives are not. In the absence of sun exposure, people in cold climates are not receiving adequate amounts of vitamin D from their skin.

- People who are taking drugs that deplete key nutrients required for various biological functions. (See Chapter 11.)

- Nutritionally-related SNPs that predispose people to being deficient in key vitamins and minerals (as you learned in Chapter 5).

- Anyone who believes in the concept of optimal well-being and rejects being "normal." It's normal to eat SAD, and normal for almost half of the country to be overweight or obese, but it sure isn't optimal.

- Women with life-stage needs. People with chronic diseases. The elderly. The very young. Growing teens. Athletes. All the groups with special nutritional needs, including vegetarians who tend to be low in B12, iron, and zinc.

I will pause my tirade briefly and note one thing the speaker did get right. People taking excessive quantities of water-soluble B vitamins and vitamin C pee out the excess, hence the reference to expense.

But back to my rant: It's so easy to make generalizations or to divide the world into "everyone" or "no one." In this case, the presenter used "vitamins" as the catch-all phrase to refer to all supplements. Hey, what about macro and microminerals? What about the healing power of herbs? Did he not realize that, according to the US Forest Service, "A full 40 percent of the drugs behind the pharmacist's counter in the Western world are derived from plants that people have used for centuries, including the top 20 best-selling prescription drugs in the United States today." This would include drugs like aspirin, derived from willow bark, or digitalis derived from the foxglove plant, or a drug like penicillin that originated from a mold.[118]

While I can conjure up even more questions I wished I had asked, there's only one that's spot on for you: Are *you* taking the *right* supplements to create healthy glowing skin?

Dietary Supplements Right or Wrong

The right supplement is, first and foremost, a high quality and safe product, free from impurities or toxins. Companies that produce high-quality nutraceuticals follow a set of manufacturing guidelines known as certified good manufacturing practices (cGMP) established by the US Food and Drug Administration (FDA). cGMP dictates how domestic and foreign companies manufacture, package, label, and sell dietary supplements in the United States.[119]

The cGMPs cover a lot more than just basic hygienic practices pertaining to employees, manufacturing equipment, and the physical plant. There are also quality control measures, oversight procedures, corrective action plans, and data tracking and reporting requirements. Raw materials, especially those of plant origin, must be properly sourced, identified, validated, and processed. The cGMPs, when followed, means that the supplement manufacturer can answer what the ingredient is, where it came from, how pure it is, and how it was processed. When cGMPs are followed, the consumer can have confidence that the supplement they're taking is efficacious and safe. Furthermore, the best companies routinely undergo third party certification and validation to make certain that what they claim on the label (such as, 100 mg of substance X) is the amount of active ingredient in the product.

Manufacturing features and third-party certifications may include:

- Certified Organic
- Vegan
- Vegetarian
- Certified Kosher
- Halal Certified
- Non-GMO Project Verified
- Dairy & Soy Free
- Glyphosate Residue Free
- Tested for Herbs & Pesticides

POTENTIAL ISSUES WITH PLANT-BASED INGREDIENTS OR BOTANICAL EXTRACTS

- Incorrect identification of plant source (it's not what it's supposed to be)
- Adulteration with a different plant species (another plant species is mixed in)
- Environmental contaminants (pesticide/herbicide residues, heavy metals)
- Biological contaminants (microbes, toxins produced by prior infestation)

The Supplement World is Divided into Two Camps

So how do you know if your supplement is safe and effective? Companies that sell to the professional healthcare channel check all the boxes for quality and safety noted above. You will always be best served by obtaining your supplements from a nutrition-oriented professional. No matter how well you educate yourself, nothing compares to obtaining guidance from a clinician who can use your medical history, a physical exam, and laboratory tests to personalize your treatment plan.

Many consumers who visit a functional medicine practitioner, and are prescribed professional grade products, are tempted to buy similar over-the-counter supplements to save money. This creates problems for the practitioner in terms of determining what's working. Shilpa Saxena, MD, Chief Medical Officer & Physician at Forum Health, LLC, describes the issue this way:

> "I always remind patients what happens if they choose a supplement brand with which I have no experience. If they don't get the desired result, we are left to wonder two things. Was this the wrong nutrient? Or was this the wrong brand? It's unnecessarily more complicated, at times, and usually more costly for the patient in the long run."

Increasingly for patient convenience, more and more healthcare professionals are offering online nutritional formularies for their patients. In this case, the formulary manager—usually Fullscript, or Wellevate from Emerson Ecologics—vets the quality of the product, and fulfills the product directly to the patient. The professional channel companies with whom I have the greatest familiarity are listed below. Many of the products from these companies can also be found online.

PROFESSIONAL CHANNEL COMPANIES	
Allergy Research Group®	Metagenics®
American River™ Nutrition	OrthoMolecular Products®
Apex Energetics™	Pure Encapsulations®
Biotics Research®	Quicksilver Scientific

Designs for Health®	Sovereign Laboratories™
Douglas Laboratories®	Standard Process®
Enzyme Science™	Thorne®
Integrative Therapeutics®	Vital Nutrients
Klaire Labs®	Xymogen®

How do You Know the Supplement Works?

The DSHEA act, passed in 1994, defines and regulates dietary supplements. It specifically sets out a separate regulatory process for supplements (as opposed to regulating them like pharmaceutical drugs). Manufacturers and distributors of dietary supplements are prohibited from making drug claims which involve preventing or treating a disease. So, a supplement company can't say their supplement "prevents or treats COVID-19 infection." They *can* state a structure-function claim, describing how the supplement works. For example, a supplement company can say that a certain supplement "supports immune health" or "supports healthy collagen and elastin."

However, the manufacturer or distributor must have evidence on file to support this. These structure and function claims are regulated by the FTC; the FDA only gets involved when the manufacturer steps over the line and makes a drug claim. The FDA can also investigate violations of cGMP manufacturing.

Studies to support dietary supplement structure and function may be performed in the laboratory, on animals, or on humans. Human studies are usually small, involving anywhere from a few dozen to a few hundred subjects. The studies are often conducted by the company which manufactures the active ingredient: formulators or distributors of supplements that use the active ingredient can then rely on these studies for their own claims.

In medicine, we are always seeking evidence, the best form of which is a randomized clinical trial (RCT). In an RCT, there is a control group taking a placebo, in addition to the group receiving the "real" treatment. Both the patients and the investigators may be "blinded," so that neither knows whether the study participant is taking the supplement or a placebo.

For supplements, the more professional companies will do a clinical study, often an RTC, on their final formulated product in humans. For skin beauty, the studies seek to prove a certain endpoint—such as improvement in skin elasticity, barrier protection, reduction in acne lesion counts, redness, or pigment. Professional companies spend more time and money to gather the evidence in a way that is acceptable to doctors; this is often the reason that the products are premium-priced.

Direct-to-Consumer Dietary Supplements

There are two major consumer distribution channels: retail and online. Consumers today can purchase supplements at their grocery, pharmacy, or specialty retailer. Increasingly, people are going online to buy. In either case, the number of choices is often bewildering. How do you know if you are buying a quality supplement in a store or online?

To answer this question, I turned to Tom Aarts, who founded and runs the Nutrition Business Summit, a meeting of the top supplement companies in the world. I asked Tom, point blank, which consumer companies he had the most trust in. While he noted that many of the smaller companies produce quality products, the companies he felt comfortable recommending (in alphabetic order) include:

Enzymedica® enzymedica.com	Committed to being carbon neutral, supports people and planet, rigorous testing
Garden of Life® gardenoflife.com	Preach and follow through on their commitment to quality, purity, and safety
MegaFood® megafood.com	Emphasize "farm fresh" ingredients; feature multiple certifications
New Chapter® newchapter.com	Ferment vitamins for greater absorption, emphasis on sustainable sourcing
Now Foods® nowfoods.com	Tend to be the low-cost leader with solid inhouse testing
Rainbow Light® rainbowlight.com	Great tasting gummies, as well as a diverse line of multivitamins

Test First

There are three things that really bother me about the current business and practice of supplement use. The first is the mistaken equivalence between supplements and food. Supplements are not food; they only fill in for insufficiencies. They are no substitute for a crappy diet. The second is the misguided belief that, because a person is taking boatloads of supplements, they are somehow immune from getting ill. It is true that nutrition coupled with intelligent supplement use can help people stay healthier, and if they do become ill, recover faster. However, pills, powders, liquids, and gummies are not magic bullets. They don't come with an illness-free guarantee. The third issue I have is that most people don't get the proper laboratory tests to determine what their body needs and how they can track and monitor progress. The most common nutrition-related laboratory tests—obtainable from most standard labs—will measure vitamin and mineral levels in addition to a complete blood count and a basic metabolic panel.

Open Wide and Say Ahhh…

Technology has changed the practice of medicine—one of the negatives of this shift is that it has relegated the physical exam to the back seat. Yet, when it comes to identifying nutritional deficiencies, the first place to look is the mouth and tongue. Why? Because, according to Functional Medicine physician Michael Stone, MD, of Ashland Oregon, these tissues have the fastest turnover in the body. Stone teaches the nutrition-oriented physical exam to clinicians who attend trainings at The Institute for Functional Medicine (IFM.org). According to Stone, an astute physician—or an equally smart consumer—can find signs of vitamin and mineral deficiency before laboratory findings identify the problem.

Color and texture are two prime indicators of nutritional health. If your tongue is purplish-blue, this may indicate a vitamin B2 deficiency (or you could have eaten a bunch of blueberries). A beefy-red and glossy tongue could signal a vitamin B12 deficiency. Iron deficiency often results in a pale-colored tongue. Advanced vitamin B or vitamin A deficiencies can cause cracks and fissures which cover the surface of the tongue in what is sometimes called "geographic tongue." The surface looks like a topography map; it may also be accompanied by a separate, but concurrent oral yeast infection. (I'm guessing now is the time you're setting this book down and heading for the bathroom mirror.)

The visual signs and painful symptoms of micronutrient deficiencies can be indicative of other serious situations unrelated to nutritional intake and absorption, so be sure to check with your primary care provider regardless. Here are some of the most common vitamin deficiency-induced tongue conditions:

- **Smooth Tongue**
  An abnormally smooth, inflamed, and red-colored tongue is called "atrophic glossitis," or simply "glossitis," and it results when the papillae (tiny, fingerlike projections on the tongue) disappear. Glossitis is caused by an ongoing deficiency of one or more vitamins from the B family—folate, vitamin B12, or niacin. Vegans, patients with Crohn's and other digestive diseases, and alcoholics are prone to getting glossitis. Reversing the deficiency with supplementation is typically sufficient to return the tongue to its normal state. The papillae grow back rapidly once the deficiency is corrected.

- **Fissured Tongue**
  A tongue with deep fissures or grooves can be the result of a vitamin A deficiency or advanced vitamin B deficiency. The fissures can collect harmful bacteria, so keeping the tongue clean by brushing or tongue scraping is important. Vitamin A deficiency is relatively rare but can be triggered by malabsorptive conditions such as celiac disease, cystic fibrosis, and cirrhosis. Vitamin supplementation is recommended once blood tests confirm the specific vitamin deficiency. Fissured tongue is also common in patients with psoriasis or Sjogren syndrome, two autoimmune diseases that affect connective tissue.

- **Ulcerated Tongue**
  Painful, bleeding ulcers on the tongue, lips, throat, and inside of the cheeks result from severe vitamin C deficiency (scurvy); these are referred to as "scurvy ulcers." In some people, the ulcers do not bleed but are covered by a thick, gray membrane. Niacin (vitamin B3) deficiency can also cause a red tongue and mouth pain, progressing to ulcers under the tongue and lower lip, which then appear throughout the mouth; bleeding and more intense pain follows.

- **Burning Tongue**
  A burning or tingling sensation in the tongue can stem from a vitamin B deficiency, especially vitamin B12, and iron deficiency.[120]

Laboratory Testing

If there is a fluid in the body, there's a way to test it. While hair can be used to check for toxic quantities of heavy metals, and saliva and swabs assess for genes, the most actionable nutrition information can be found from simple blood tests. When it comes to lab tests, you've got two basic choices: venipuncture (drawing blood from a vein) or finger-prick. The advantage of drawing blood from a vein is the amount of blood you can obtain. The more blood or serum (blood without the red cells) collected, the more tests that can be performed. In comparison, finger-pricks yield only a few drops of blood; hence, the number of tests will be limited. Often the blood from the fingerstick is applied to a strip that safely dries the blood for later analysis.

In order to get a blood draw, you can either go through your doctor, or you can order directly from a company that uses the same standard certified laboratories used by physicians. I have had excellent service from Ulta Lab Tests. They offer panels of tests for various conditions, including a group of tests that measure the key vitamins and minerals involved in skin health. All you need to do is go online, fill out some information, and then you will be directed to print out a form which you'll take to Quest Laboratories. Once you've made an appointment and had your blood drawn, the results are uploaded into a secure online portal and you are notified by email as soon as they're available. The specific skin-health related tests they make available are shown below.

The Ulta Lab Test Skin Health Vitamin and Minerals Panel

- Calcium
- Copper
- Magnesium, RBC
- Omega-3 and -6 Fatty Acids, Plasma
- QuestAssureD™ 25-Hydroxyvitamin D (D2, D3)
- Vitamin B12 (Cobalamin) and Folate Panel, Serum
- Zinc
- Selenium

Menstruating Women

- Ferritin
- Iron and Total Iron Binding Capacity (TIBC)

Suspected Insulin Resistance

- Hemoglobin A1c
- Glucose
- Insulin

IgE Food Allergy Panel (14 biomarkers)

- Almond
- Cashew Nut
- Codfish
- Cow's Milk
- Egg White
- Hazelnut
- Peanut
- Salmon
- Scallop
- Sesame Seed
- Shrimp
- Soybean
- Tuna
- Walnut

> While Ulta Lab Tests already offers significant discounts, they have created an additional special discount for *FYSR* readers. You'll find ordering instructions for the tests as well as the additional discounts at ultalabtests.com/FYSR.

Finger-Prick Plus and Minuses

I like the convenience of being able to monitor my vitamin D level and my ratio of omega-6/omega-3 from a simple one-drop of blood. You can obtain both tests from Omegaquant.com, and if you use the code "FYSR," there's an additional savings above their normal low price. Laboratories that have traditionally only served the professional market, such as ZRT Laboratory, are going direct to consumers. Increasingly, consumer-facing laboratory companies such as Let's Get Checked (letsgetchecked.com) or Everlywell (everlywell.com) are creating panels of tests which they are aggressively marketing to consumers.

For patients who want to use the convenience of a fingerstick to obtain multiple tests, but have difficulty obtaining enough blood, there are practitioners who will draw the blood with a venipuncture and then mete out the drops of blood in the collection kit.

Regardless of where you get your testing done, it is always a good idea to bring the lab results to a trusted functional medicine clinician who can sync up the labs with your health history and physical exam and help you create a personalized treatment plan. Yes, there is more cost up front, but in the long run you may save money (to say nothing of getting better results) by avoiding the *DIY* approach. Your clinician can help you understand what supplements to take together to boost absorption (such as curcumin, fish oils, and vitamin D); what supplements should not be taken in tandem; when to take the supplements; and what ratios of minerals are most effective for health.

The Bottom Line

Before we move on and discuss how the various vitamins and minerals work to create skin beauty, let's just revisit my recommendations. Namely, you can't go wrong if you stick with any of the supplement manufacturers in this chapter. Self-observation is critical for health, so stick out your tongue and take a look. Finally, it's always best to test whenever you can so that you can get a baseline and monitor your progress.

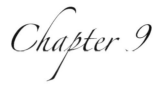

Chapter 9

VITAMINS & MINERALS FOR SKIN HEALTH & BEAUTY

Vitamins and minerals are considered essential micronutrients—because acting together, they perform hundreds of critical functions in the body. They help fuel the mitochondria that provide energy for the cells. They strengthen and protect cell membranes. They bolster the immune system. They convert food into energy. They repair cellular damage done to the skin. In this chapter, we'll explore the role that these oral vitamins and minerals play in skin health and beauty.

When it comes to supplements, we all want to know the same things. How much should I take? Is it possible to take too little, or too much?

The Vitamin & Mineral Spectrum

It's helpful to think of nutrient requirements on a *spectrum*. On the far left, we have frank *deficiency* with signs and symptoms of too few vitamins or minerals. Unless you have a serious medical condition, it's very rare for most Americans to demonstrate nutrition-deficiency disease. Just a bit to the right, there's *adequacy*, the amount that most people are getting from diet alone that prevents obvious nutrition-related disease. Then there's the sweet spot, the *optimal* amount for you (based upon your diet, genetics, medication use, and other personalized factors). Finally, there's *excess*, the amount of nutrient that can lead to signs and symptoms of overuse.

> **THE VITAMIN/MINERAL SPECTRUM**
> DEFICIENT ▶ ADEQUATE ▶ OPTIMAL ▶ EXCESS

In general, higher levels of the water-soluble vitamins are harmless, with the excess excreted in the urine. Fat soluble vitamins can accumulate in the liver; hence you should avoid excessive excess consumption.

The Alphabet Soup of Good Nutrition

Throughout this book, I have referred to RDAs—Recommended Daily Allowances. The RDAs, to remind, are a guide set forth by the US government to help us know what and how much to eat in order to be "healthy." If you are already familiar with this term, you probably recognize it from the back of your food cartons—listing out percentages of specific nutrients in foods and packaged products. But unless you're a dietitian or a nutritional scientist, you probably have no idea (and you may not care) that there's a whole bunch of other RDA-related terminology—AI, UL, EAR, DRI.[121] While you do not need to become conversant in these other acronyms, you may find them useful—so I've broken down the most important terms below.

THE ALPHABET SOUP OF GOOD NUTRITION

RDA: Recommended Dietary (or Daily) Allowance is the average daily dietary intake level that is sufficient to meet the nutrient requirement of nearly all (97 to 98 percent) healthy individuals in a group.

AI: Adequate Intake is the best estimate quantity of a specific nutrient for healthy individuals when there is insufficient research to establish an RDA.

UL: Tolerable Upper Intake Limit the highest level of daily nutrient intake that is likely to pose no risk of adverse health effects to almost all individuals in the general population. As intake increases above the UL, the risk of adverse effects increases.

EAR: Estimated Average Requirement is the quantity of a specific nutrient that is estimated to meet the nutritional requirement of one half of healthy individuals in a group.

DRI: Dietary Reference Intake is a set of values for the nutrient intakes, and it includes the Recommended Dietary Allowance (RDA), the Adequate Intake (AI), the Tolerable Upper Limit (TUL), and the Estimated Average Requirement (EAR); DRI has replaced the RDA.

In the text that follows, I note the RDA guidelines where appropriate—or interesting. You'll find additional information on nutrient deficiency and excessive consumption in Appendix B.

WATER-SOLUBLE VITAMINS

These types of vitamins, as with fat-soluble vitamins, are considered organic compounds, meaning that they can be broken down by heat, air, or acid. The water-soluble variety specifically dissolves in water. Once digested (food sources) or dissolved (supplements) in the liquid environment of the stomach and small intestine, these vitamins are absorbed into the bloodstream and transported to the body's tissues. If more of a particular water-soluble vitamin is taken into the body than what the body uses, the excess is excreted in the urine.

Water-soluble vitamins include the B-Complex and vitamin C. The ones most impactful to skin health and beauty include folate, vitamin B6, vitamin B12, and vitamin C.

BIOTIN (Vitamin B7)
Biotin is necessary for the metabolism of proteins (amino acids), glucose, and fatty acids. It also plays a role in communication between cells and gene regulation. High-biotin foods include beef liver and other organ meats, meat, fish, eggs, almonds, sunflower seeds, and sweet potatoes. Some food processing methods such as canning can reduce biotin content, so for maximum biotin, eat whole and unprocessed sources. Sole biotin supplements are available to consumers, as are B-complex supplements and "hair and nail strengthening" formulas which contain upwards of 1667-3334% of the RDA.

Despite the popularity and prevalence of biotin in hair and nail supplements, there is not a lot of science supporting its efficacy.[122,123] Biotin deficiency is extremely rare because the gut microbiota produce more biotin than what the body needs. Furthermore, severe biotin deficiency has never been documented in healthy individuals who eat a normal, varied diet.[124] Some individuals may have a biotin inadequacy due to either a very rare enzyme deficiency or alcoholism.[125,126] Biotin is an important B vitamin; however, until there is better data, I caution people to have reasonable expectations of what it can and can't do in larger doses.

FOLATE (Folic acid, Vitamin B9)
Folate functions as a coenzyme in the metabolism of nucleic and amino acids and is important during periods of rapid cell division and growth such as pregnancy. Folic acid is the synthetic version of folate and can be

obtained via supplements and fortified foods. Natural sources of folate include leafy green vegetables (spinach and turnip greens), asparagus, Brussels sprouts, citrus fruits and juices, dried beans and black-eyed peas, and beef liver.

Skin Benefits of Folate
- **Improves skin's appearance and texture.** Folate increases skin firmness by helping produce new skin cells and contributing to collagen production. Folate works against skin discoloration and may help address vitiligo (whitish skin patches where melanin is depleted).
- **Encourages hair growth.** Folate renews the cells involved in hair growth and may prevent age-related thinning of the hair if the individual is folate-deficient. Folate deficiency is also suspected in premature greying of the hair.
- **Plays a role in skin cancer.** Getting the RDA of folate may be protective against UV damage to skin cells and reduce the risk of skin cancer, but getting too much folate could possibly increase the risk of developing skin cancer.[127]
- **Improves inflammatory skin conditions.** Correcting a folate deficiency helps lower homocysteine levels in the blood, a contributing factor to chronic plaque psoriasis.

VITAMIN B6
The active form of vitamin B6 is pyridoxal 5'-phosphate which functions as a coenzyme in nearly 200 metabolic reactions involving amino acids and proteins, glucose, and lipids. Vitamin B6 is also involved in immune function, the formation of hemoglobin, neurotransmitter synthesis for cognitive development, and maintaining normal homocysteine levels in the blood. Foods with the most vitamin B6 include meats (particularly beef liver and other organ meats), fish, starchy vegetables, canned chickpeas, bananas, whole grains (highest concentration is in the germ), and nuts. Pyridoxine is the form commonly found in supplements.

Skin Benefits of Vitamin B6
- **Relieves skin conditions.** Vitamin B6 helps relieve dry skin, dermatitis, and eczema. Correcting a vitamin B6 deficiency helps reduce homocysteine levels which may help improve inflammatory-

related conditions such as chronic plaque psoriasis. Acne-prone patients may benefit by supplementing up to the tolerable upper intake level because vitamin B6 helps reduce sebum production.
- **Improves skin's appearance via detoxification.** Vitamin B6 helps the liver remove chemical toxins from the body for glowing, healthy-looking skin.

VITAMIN B12

Vitamin B12 is one of the more important vitamins in terms of human health, and its two active forms are methylcobalamin and 5-deoxyadenosylcobalamin. These and other forms of vitamin B12 contain the mineral cobalt, hence the term "cobalamins," which refers to compounds with vitamin B12 activity. Vitamin B12 is essential to optimal neurological function, proper formation of red blood cells, DNA synthesis, and protein and fat metabolism.

B12 plays an important role in the conversion of homocysteine to methionine; in doing so, it lowers homocysteine levels. Homocysteine is an amino acid naturally present in blood, but elevated levels (hyperhomocysteinemia) lead to inflammation in blood vessels, thereby increasing the risk of coronary heart disease.

Absorption of vitamin B12 is dependent on both the amount in foods, and the body's ability to produce hydrochloric acid, which drives digestion. Vitamin B12 is found in lots of different foods, but only in animal sources—not plant sources. Beef liver and clams are top of the list, followed by fish, meat, eggs, milk, and milk products. Breakfast cereals are typically fortified, as are nutritional yeasts, but the amount of this fortification is not normally enough to sustain a vegetarian's needs. Vegans are at a significant disadvantage when it comes to vitamin B12, so supplements are necessary to prevent deficiency and poor health. Any woman following a vegetarian or vegan diet during pregnancy or breastfeeding should consult with her doctor or pediatrician about supplementation.

Skin Benefits of Vitamin B12
- **Improves inflammatory skin conditions.** Correcting a vitamin B12 deficiency helps lower homocysteine levels in the blood, a contributing factor to chronic plaque psoriasis.

A word of caution. Some research has shown that injectable vitamin B12 ("vitamin B-12 shots") can change the genetic expression of the bacteria in the skin's pores (*Propionibacterium acnes*) and cause it to produce inflammatory substances called porphyrins.[128] Oral supplementation of vitamin B12 rarely has the same effect but may promote breakouts in acne-prone individuals. Vitamin B12 IV drips, which have become popular in medspas, should be used with caution in people with significant acne.

VITAMIN C

L-ascorbic acid is the functional form of vitamin C which works as a powerful antioxidant and is necessary for various biological reactions within the body. Ascorbic acid is an electron donor for enzymes which help stabilize the structure of collagen and synthesize carnitine, amino acids, and hormones. Carnitine is significant because it assists the mitochondria by transporting fatty acids into them for energy production and by removing cellular waste from cells. The human body cannot manufacture its own vitamin C, so we must get it from dietary sources, of which the most abundant include orange and grapefruit juice, papayas, peaches, and sweet red peppers.

Skin Benefits of Vitamin C

- **Improves skin's firmness.** Vitamin C contributes to healthy collagen production for firmer skin (less sagging) and fewer fine lines.
- **Improves skin's appearance.** As a potent antioxidant, vitamin C reduces skin inflammation and redness by neutralizing free radicals. It may also afford some protection against UV radiation and pre-cancerous growths.

While vitamin C performs many essential functions in the human body, depending upon the supplement formulation, limited amounts may reach the skin due to low bioavailability.[129] PureWay-C® is a formulation that is rapidly absorbed and leads to higher levels in the body. It can be found as a branded ingredient in many oral formulations. In addition, topical application of vitamin C serums is highly advantageous. I'll discuss this in greater detail later on.

FAT-SOLUBLE VITAMINS

Unlike water-soluble vitamins which easily enter the bloodstream, the fat-soluble vitamins (A, D, E, K) are relatively non-dissolvable in water and have a more complex journey. After you eat a food that contains a fat-soluble vitamin, the digestive process begins in the stomach and continues in the small intestine where bile from the liver assists in breaking down the fats. The fat-soluble vitamins are absorbed through the small intestine wall and enter the lymph vessel where they are essentially paired off with a protein "escort" before entering the bloodstream. Without the protein escort, fat-soluble vitamins would be unable to travel to the body's tissues. Any surplus is stored in the liver and body fat. If the body requires a particular fat-soluble vitamin, the liver or fat tissue receives a signal to release some from the reserve supply.

Because of this storage capacity, frank deficiencies are typically rare among Americans. Much more common are insufficiencies, and sometimes toxicities from excessive supplementation. There are many factors affecting each individual's micronutrient needs, so the ideal replenishment schedule differs among people. Blood tests to measure baseline vitamin status should be considered to check for any deficiencies or toxicities.

VITAMIN A

The term 'Vitamin A' includes a group of retinoids (retinol, retinal, retinyl esters) which play an important role in vision, immunity, reproduction, and maintaining organs including the heart, lungs, and kidneys. Retinoids do this this by supporting communication between cells and by stimulating cell growth and differentiation (i.e., the process of a stem cell developing into a more specialized type of cell). Retinal and retinoic acid are the active forms of vitamin A responsible for these biological functions, so metabolic processes within the cells must occur before vitamin A is functional. Retinol is converted to retinal and then to retinoic acid. Excess vitamin A is stored in the liver.

Foods contain one of two different types of vitamin A—preformed vitamin A (retinol, retinyl ester) and provitamin A carotenoids (beta-carotene, alpha-carotene, beta-cryptoxanthin), the plant pigments which the body converts to vitamin A. Animal foods, such as milk, eggs, meat (particularly beef liver), fish, fish oils, and fortified cereals contain preformed vitamin A. Good sources of provitamin A are leafy green vegetables, broccoli, carrots, sweet potatoes, squash, and cantaloupe; milk and eggs have smaller amounts.

Skin Benefits of Vitamin A
- **Protects against UV damage and slows signs of aging.** Vitamin A acts as a natural sunscreen by lessening the skin's sensitivity, thereby preventing redness or pigmentation. As an antioxidant, vitamin A neutralizes free radicals that otherwise break down collagen in the skin and cause it to develop fine lines or lose firmness.
- **Encourages production of new skin cells.** Vitamin A stimulates growth of new fibroblasts which maintain firmness deep within the skin's layers. This promotes stronger, more hydrated skin and efficient wound healing. Topical skin creams containing vitamin A encourage faster skin cell turnover.
- **Strengthens the skin barrier.** Vitamin A promotes regeneration of cells which strengthen the barrier from bacteria, pollution, and other skin irritants.

VITAMIN D
Calciferol is a group of chemical compounds collectively known as vitamin D; the two most relevant forms are vitamin D_2 (ergocalciferol) and vitamin D_3 (cholecalciferol). Vitamin D helps the body absorb calcium through the small intestine and ensures healthy bone mineralization by balancing adequate levels of calcium and phosphate. This is essential for bone growth and repair, as well as for preventing the formation of thin, brittle, or malformed bones. Vitamin D also contributes to reducing inflammation and promoting cell growth, glucose metabolism, immune function, and neuromuscular function.

Vitamin D_3 is photosynthesized by the skin when exposed to ultraviolet B radiation from the sun. The keratinocytes in the epidermis contain the enzymes necessary to convert vitamin D into its active form—1,25-dihydroxyvitamin D_3, which functions as a steroid hormone. Regular sun exposure generates sufficient vitamin D_3, but access to sunlight can be limited by a person's geographical location, season, amount of skin pigmentation, age, and use of sunscreens. Vitamin D is available naturally in a just a few foods, including fatty fish, fish-liver oils, beef liver, egg yolks, and mushrooms. Fortified milk products, orange juice, and breakfast cereals have vitamin D added to compensate for lack of sun exposure and natural sources in the diet.

Skin Benefits of Vitamin D
- **Maintains general skin health.** Vitamin D is involved in promoting normal skin cell growth and maintaining the integrity of the skin barrier. Skin remains youthful looking.
- **Supports wound healing & tissue repair.** Vitamin D regulates an antimicrobial protein (cathelicidin) which is believed to modulate inflammation and control immunity in the skin.
- **Protects against photoaging & skin cancer.** Topically-applied vitamin D may prevent or reduce DNA damage in the skin cells and reduce cell death caused by UV light exposure.

Because vitamin D is so important to skin health, we need to be aware of vitamin D insufficiency ("lower-than-ideal levels"), which is quite common, and now being identified by routine bloodwork. Older adults have lower levels because aging skin loses some of its vitamin D synthesizing capacity and because older people tend to stay out of the sun, especially if ill or immobilized. Also, people with darker skin have more melanin which reduces vitamin D synthesis.

VITAMIN E
'Vitamin E' collectively refers to a group of 8 naturally-occurring forms—alpha-, beta-, gamma-, and delta-tocopherol and alpha-, beta-, gamma-, and delta-tocotrienol—which function as antioxidants. As a fat-soluble antioxidant, vitamin E stops the production of free radicals (reactive oxygen species) which are otherwise created when the fat in foods is oxidized. Vitamin E also plays a role in immune function, communication between cells, regulating how certain genes get expressed, and various other metabolic processes.

The form of vitamin E that is most commonly found in supplements is alpha-tocopherol. The challenge with this form of supplement is that existing studies on oral vitamin E supplementation with alpha-tocopherol don't consistently show health or skin benefits.[130] There is some concern that vitamin E may increase the risk of prostate cancer.[131] Given the inconsistencies with alpha-tocopherol, there's a growing body of research showing that we may have been led down the wrong path with oral vitamin E supplementation.

Barrie Tan, PhD, is one of the world's foremost experts on vitamin E. He has devoted much of his adult life to studying the action of tocotrienols that are produced by the annatto plant, a shrub native to Central and South America, often called the "Lipstick tree." Dr. Tan has extracted the delta-tocotrienol component of the plant and points to multiple benefits: neuroprotective, antioxidant, and anti-inflammatory. Studies show that tocotrienol supplementation can reduce the signs of aging, decrease sun damage, and improve the ability to fight skin infections.[132,133] Furthermore, topical application may help heal wounds.[134]

Nuts, seeds, and vegetable oils are the best natural sources of vitamin E. Wheat germ oil, sunflower seeds, and almonds pack the biggest nutritional punch. Most Americans, however, get their vitamin E from soybean, canola, and corn oils, and fortified food products, which are less than ideal products to consume.

Skin Benefits of Vitamin E

- **Improves skin's appearance.** As an antioxidant, oral vitamin E neutralizes free radicals and reduces inflammation.
- **Remediates dry skin.** Oral supplementation may help counterbalance very low sebum production in the pores; sebum conditions the skin and prevents dryness under optimal conditions.
- **Protects against sun damage.** Topically-applied vitamin E absorbs skin-damaging ultraviolet light from the sun and helps prevent wrinkles and dark-colored spots. A topical product with both vitamin E and vitamin C likely offers more protection than either one alone. Dr. Tan's research has shown topical delta-tocotrienol can produce an SPF of around 5 to aid in skin protection.

VITAMIN K

'Vitamin K' collectively refers to compounds with a common structure; these include phylloquinone (vitamin K1) and several menaquinones (forms of vitamin K2). Vitamin K acts as an essential coenzyme to synthesize proteins needed for blood clotting and bone metabolism. Due to vitamin K's relationship to bone and immune health, as well as cardiovascular protection, many supplements combine K2 and D_3. Noteworthy products are manufactured by Designs for Health,

OrthoMolecular Products, Enzymedica (all plant-based), and Quicksilver Scientific (a convenient liquid spray). To get the most from these supplements, they should be taken with a meal.

Leafy green vegetables are high in vitamin K2, with turnip and collard greens, spinach, and kale having significant quantities; one serving meets or exceeds the RDA. Vitamin K2 is found in fermented foods such as natto (fermented soybeans) and cheese; the amount of vitamin K2 is influenced by which bacteria strains are used to ferment the food. The gut microbiota also produces vitamin K2—a good reason to maintain a healthy microbiome.

Skin Benefits of Vitamin K

- **Improve skin's appearance following skin injury.** Because vitamin K is essential to blood clotting and in turn, wound healing, it's likely to benefit bruising, dark-colored spots, stretch marks, and scars. This may improve recovery time after cosmetic surgery.
- **Promote surgical wound healing.** Topically-applied vitamin K is often used to reduce swelling and bruising, as well as to promote overall skin healing following surgery.

MINERALS

Unlike vitamins, minerals are inorganic compounds and retain their chemical structure when they enter the body. When we eat food or drink water, we can trace the minerals in our food back to what that food itself "ate" during its formation, alongside what environment our food was raised or grown in. That means the minerals in the soil where the plants were grown, and the plants that fed the cattle, pigs, and chicken we eat, and the little fish that become food for the bigger fish that we eventually eat. Mineral content doesn't degrade with cooking or storage, so whatever's in your food when it was harvested or butchered—that's what's in it when you put it into your mouth.

Minerals contribute to the building of strong bones and muscles and play important roles in maintaining various bodily functions. Minerals can be subdivided in to two classifications—macrominerals (major minerals) and microminerals (trace minerals). The body needs macrominerals in relatively large quantities, and a deficiency can incur health consequences. Conversely, the body needs relatively small quantities of microminerals, and ingesting excessive amounts—either from supplements or from 'contaminated' food—can induce toxicity and be deleterious to health. For most microminerals, there's a fine line between 'just enough' and 'too much.' Eating a varied diet provides an adequate and safe amount, so supplementation might be overdoing it. If you are considering exceeding the RDAs for minerals, it's a good idea to assess your levels before starting and then after three and six months to see what effects are taking place.

The most impactful minerals to skin health and beauty are calcium, copper, magnesium, potassium, selenium, and zinc. Below, I discuss each of these minerals in turn.

CALCIUM

Calcium is the body's most abundant mineral, with 99% of it stored in the bones and teeth. The other 1% circulates in the muscles, blood, and intercellular fluids, and is utilized for contraction and dilation of the blood vessels, muscle function, nerve transmission, cell-to-cell communication and hormone secretion. These functions are tightly regulated, as is the calcium needed to fuel them, so if more calcium is needed, the body takes from the bone stores. Extra calcium from the diet is transferred to the bones so that the 1:99 ratio remains consistent; it can also be excreted in sweat, urine, or feces.

High quantities of calcium are found naturally in dairy milk, yogurt, and cheese, canned sardines, and salmon (as long as you eat the bones). Kale, bok choi, and broccoli contain modest amounts, along with fortified orange juice, soy milk, tofu, and breakfast cereals. On average, 30% of the calcium in foods is absorbed by the body.

Skin Benefits of Calcium

- **Promotes new skin cell growth.** Calcium helps regulate the rate of skin cell turnover. Skin may appear thin or dry if there are insufficient calcium stores.
- **Helps retain skin's moisture.** Calcium facilitates sebum production in the epidermis which naturally helps the skin retain moisture.
- **Helps prevent skin cancer.** Calcium helps regulate skin cells that contain melanin; this gives rise to tanned skin that is protected from harmful UV rays.

COPPER

Functioning as a cofactor for numerous enzymes, copper is essential to the body's ability to produce energy, synthesize neurotransmitters, metabolize iron, and synthesize connective tissue. It also plays a role in optimal immune system function, brain development, gene regulation, new blood vessel development, and skin pigmentation. The body stores only small amounts of copper in muscle and skeletal tissue. Copper absorption in the small intestine is influenced by how much copper is actually in the diet; more is absorbed if the diet is low in copper, and less is absorbed if the diet is high in copper.

Beef liver, wild oysters, and chocolate are the richest dietary sources, followed by other shellfish, nuts, seeds, potatoes (and their skins), mushrooms, and whole-grain products. Tap water is also a source of copper. The amount depends on the type of water pipes supplying the home, as well as the amount in the municipal water itself.

Skin Benefits of Copper

- **Promotes youthful appearance.** Copper is involved in collagen and elastin production[135] and new blood vessel growth which helps maintain the skin's elasticity and firmness. Proteins with copper attached (GHK-cu copper peptides) act as transport mechanisms to bring restorative proteins to the skin to generate healthy new cells.[136]
- **Helps maintain skin's moisture.** Copper promotes the production of hyaluronic acid, which in turn, maintains the skin's moisture and boosts collagen production.
- **Protects against photoaging.** As an antioxidant, copper helps neutralize free radicals which otherwise attack skin cells. This helps combat the oxidative stress from UV exposure, a common cause of fine lines, wrinkles, and crepey skin.

MAGNESIUM

Magnesium is abundant in the human body and tightly regulated, with 50-60% stored in the bones, 1% in the blood, and the remainder stored in soft tissues. Magnesium functions as a cofactor in more than 300 enzymatic processes that in turn regulate major biochemical reactions that are critical to life. These include protein synthesis, energy production, blood glucose metabolism, nerve and muscle function, blood pressure regulation, bone development, DNA, RNA, glutathione synthesis, and calcium-potassium ion transport—necessary for proper nerve conduction, normal heart rhythm and healthy muscle contraction.

Magnesium is present in a wide range of foods that also contain fiber. Good sources include seeds (pumpkin and chia), nuts (almonds, cashews, and peanuts), legumes, spinach and other leafy green vegetables, and whole grains. Breakfast cereals are typically fortified with magnesium. Mineral, bottled, and tap waters contain varying amounts depending on the source and whether minerals have been added. Between 30% and 40% of dietary magnesium consumed will end up being absorbed by the body. Magnesium is often a component of laxatives and antacids.

Skin Benefits of Magnesium

- **Improves skin texture and appearance.** Bathing in a Dead Sea salt solution which is high in magnesium improves the skin's natural barrier function, increases hydration, and reduces inflammation and skin roughness.[137]
- **Relieves atopic dermatitis-associated dryness.** Topical application of a magnesium and ceramide cream improves skin hydration in patients with mild to moderate atopic dermatitis better than traditional treatments (hydrocortisone and emollient).[138]
- **Helps the underlying causes of acne.** Increased cortisol levels, resulting from stress and anxiety, can worsen acne. Magnesium helps dampen the effects of cortisol and promotes relaxation to ensure a good night's sleep.

Transdermal absorption of magnesium has been suggested as a way to increase magnesium in the body without causing the gastric upset or laxative effect that some people experience. However, most research has not found this to be true, or has found only a slight increase.[139] Yet, bathing in Dead Sea salts with magnesium is wonderful for the mind (and skin) as you relax and let your stress melt away.

WHICH MAGNESIUM SUPPLEMENT IS BEST?

If your primary care doctor or integrative practitioner has told you that your magnesium levels are lower than ideal and that you should take a supplement, chances are that they did not recommend a specific type. Not all magnesium supplements are created equal, and four forms available today seem to have the best performance—magnesium diglycinate, magnesium bisglycinate, magnesium taurate, and magnesium acetyl taurine. My top choices are either the taurate or acetyl taurine forms because of their ability to penetrate the blood-brain barrier and help improve concentration and focus.

POTASSIUM

Normal cell function depends on potassium, and so it is ubiquitous to all the body's tissues. Electrolytes—potassium and sodium—function in tandem to ensure proper nerve transmission, kidney function, and muscle contraction, including heart contractions. Fruits, especially bananas, vegetables, and some legumes are the best sources of potassium; these are present in the forms of potassium phosphate, potassium sulfate, and potassium citrate. Protein-based foods, including nuts, dairy products, meat, poultry, and fish, contain potassium in much smaller quantities. Salt substitutes contain potassium chloride which replaces all or a portion of the sodium chloride for people on salt-restricted diets. The body is capable of absorbing 85-90% of ingested potassium.

Skin Benefits of Potassium
- **Helps alleviate dry skin.** Getting enough potassium from foods is key to preventing skin from becoming severely dehydrated and hardened (xeroderma).

SELENIUM

Selenium is a component of at least two dozen selenoproteins which are essential to DNA synthesis, thyroid hormone metabolism, reproduction, and protecting the body's cells and tissues from oxidative damage and infection. Soil contains inorganic selenium which plants store and convert to organic selenium. Most of the body's selenium is stored in skeletal muscles. The amount of selenium in plant-based foods varies greatly by the soil conditions in which the plants are grown. The best source of selenium, by far, is the Brazil nut. Fish, shrimp, organ meats, and muscle meats are also rich in selenium.

Skin Benefits of Selenium
- **Helps prevent wrinkles.** As an antioxidant, oral selenium neutralizes free radicals. It works with vitamin E to protect and maintain the cell membranes of skin cells.
- **Reduces skin inflammation.** Oral selenium is likely to decrease production of inflammatory cytokines and help prevent collagen breakdown.
- **Protects against skin infections.** Oral selenium and other minerals assist the white blood cells that fight topical infections.

Getting too much selenium over a long period of time—either from foods or supplements—can result in hair and nail brittleness or loss, a condition attributed to selenosis. Most Americans don't need to worry about a deficiency.[140]

ZINC

Zinc has a critical role in cellular metabolism and is necessary for about 300 enzymatic reactions. Zinc assists in cell division, DNA synthesis, protein synthesis, immune function, and wound healing. It's also a must for your sense of smell and taste. Food sources with a high zinc content include oysters (#1), red meat, poultry, crab, lobster, beans, nuts, dairy products, whole-grain breads, and fortified breakfast cereals. Zinc from animal foods is readily absorbed by the body, but absorption of zinc in plant foods is somewhat inhibited by the phytates found naturally in grains, legumes, and other plant-based foods. Phytates bind to zinc, thereby inhibiting absorption.

Skin Benefits of Zinc

- **Helps reduce inflammation.** Oral zinc helps decrease the severity of acne and skin rashes. Lowering inflammations also helps reduce early signs of aging skin—fine lines, wrinkles, and dark-colored spots.
- **Keeps skin bacteria under control.** Zinc helps keep *Cutibacterium acnes* under control.[141] Patients with acne tend to have much lower serum zinc levels than people without acne.[142]
- **Involved with collagen synthesis.** As an enzyme cofactor, oral zinc contributes to collagen synthesis and DNA repair.
- **Helps in wound healing.** Oral and topically-applied zinc helps the healing of skin lesions and rashes. Zinc's antibacterial properties help prevent skin infections.
- **Protects against UV damage.** Topical zinc oxide acts a physical barrier and reflects the sun's damaging UV rays.

SILICON

Silicon (not to be confused with silicone) is the second most abundant element on the planet and the third most abundant trace mineral in the body. Despite being so prevalent in the body and the environment, silicon's function is less than well-established. It does however, have medicinal uses in the treatment of heart disease, osteoporosis, and aging skin. Water (plain and mineral), red wine, beer, coffee, cereals, raisins, bananas, brown rice, root vegetables, spinach, green beans, seafood, and some organ meats naturally contain silicon. So, by virtue of drinking water or coffee (or the various alcoholic beverages) every day, you're probably getting enough silicon.

The most promising form of silicon is orthosilicic acid (OSA) and choline-stabilized OSA (ch-OSA) which is approved for human consumption; it also happens that ch-OSA is the most bioavailable form of silicon. Orthosilicic acid supplements are usually made from a bamboo extract.

Skin Benefits of Silicon

- **Helps improve skin strength and elasticity.** Oral silicon helps collagen synthesis and activates enzymes.[143]
- **Helps improve hair and nail health.** Supplemental use of ch-OSA slows the rate of hair loss, reduces breakage, increases luster,[144] and improves soft or brittle nails. Individuals with low silicon levels tend to have more nail infections.

How do You Measure Up?

So now that you know which vitamins and minerals play a role in great looking skin, how does your diet measure up? A varied intake of vegetables, fruits, whole-grains, lean proteins and healthy fats is sufficient for most people to gain adequate amounts. Certain health conditions or medication use may compromise micronutrient absorption in the body, so getting baseline bloodwork done is advisable to correct any chronic deficiencies. No one wants any surprises, but if your doctor or dietitian does find an insufficiency (or toxicity), be sure to follow their nutritional guidance.

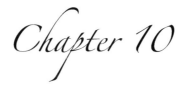

Chapter 10

BOTANICALS & BEYOND

Now that scientists have figured out a way to extract nutrients from various foods, supplement manufacturers have found a way to put them into softgels, capsules, pills, and gummies (and then into plastic bottles and glass containers). Some of these nutrients are derived from plants (botanicals and phytonutrients) while others have come from non-plant sources such as those derived from marine (fish, crustacean) or bovine (cow) sources. If you adhere to specific dietary restrictions, I encourage you to do your research when selecting supplements. Additionally, vegans, in particular, should read labels to confirm that the capsule ("veggie cap") is not made from animal sources.

It's safe to make the assumption that most supplements do not have side effects when you take them according to the manufacturer's directions. That being said, some people react differently—so be on the lookout for any sign that it's not agreeing with you. More often than not, the unpleasant or adverse symptoms will be GI-related, such as tummy upset, abdominal cramping, gas, diarrhea or constipation. This can usually be resolved by limiting the dose or discontinuing the supplement entirely. If you are pregnant or breastfeeding, you should check with your OB/GYN before taking any new supplement just to be sure.

ANTIOXIDANTS

¿Cuál es más fuerte?

When it comes to botanical antioxidants, there's always a running debate as to which are the most powerful for either general health, skin beauty, or both. The following are the key botanical supplements that convey antioxidant protection for skin.

Astaxanthin. This is one of the carotenoids that imparts the red color to certain algae. It is also responsible for the pink-red color in salmon and the red outer shell of lobsters and crabs. According to one scientific report, astaxanthin has the "highest antioxidant activity when compared to other antioxidants such as lycopene, vitamin E, and vitamin A and is usually referred to as king of antioxidants."[145]

Astaxanthin is usually available in quantities of 4 mg, 8 mg, 10 mg or 12 mg. It is often included in skin beauty formulations that include other carotenoids, as well as products that counter muscle loss with aging (sarcopenia).[146] Astaxanthin is one of the main antioxidants in my favorite daily skin drink Aethern® (aethern.com), which offers a "healthy skin from within" approach.

Lutein and zeaxanthin (L/Z). These carotenoids are commonly known as the "eye health" vitamins for their use in slowing the progression of age-related macular degeneration (AMD). Combinations of vitamins C and E, lutein, zeaxanthin, zinc, and copper may slow AMD-related vision loss.[147]

Research suggests that these supplements (made from marigold flower extract) are exceedingly valuable for the skin's overall appearance as well as protection from sun exposure. Carotenoids in general encourage skin repair and healing and protect the skin from oxidative stress and free radicals, thereby reducing the risk of some types of skin cancer.[148] Daily L/Z supplementation for just 12 weeks was shown to improve the skin's appearance and lightened skin tone.[149] In one study, oral supplementation and topical application of a L/Z serum improved hydration and reduced facial wrinkles.[150] It's highly probable that a combination of diet, oral supplementation, and topical application of these two nutrients is most advantageous for skin health, and something I feel comfortable in recommending—even in the absence of RDAs (at the present time).

The nutrients in supplements target more than one organ. For both eye and skin health, I recommend—and personally take—Eye Shield from Biological Essentials (available from amazon.com).

Lycopene
Currently, there is no RDA for lycopene. One assumption may be that consuming the Standard American Diet—chock-full of tomato-based foods (i.e., ketchup, spaghetti sauce, pizza sauce)—is sufficient. However, the processed, high-glycemic carbohydrates and sugars that go along with the lycopene-rich tomato products will fail the skin. A lycopene supplement may be the better choice; these are available in the form of

softgels and gummies. More recently, powdered lycopene extracts are being utilized as ingredients added to other health foods. One such company, Lycored (lycored.com), has been on the forefront of lycopene and skin research since 1995, and offers their product as a branded ingredient in multiple skin formulations.

OTHER NOTEWORTHY ANTIOXIDANTS

There are additional antioxidants with potentially promising effects for anti-aging and inflammatory-related skin diseases. And while much of the research is currently being done with topical applications with carrier molecules and/or in animal models, taking these supplements orally allows the nutrient to travel through the bloodstream and enter the dermis. It should be noted that some of these compounds have low oral bioavailability, yet on the whole, they act by reducing oxidative stress and inflammation to some degree. They are generally found in a varied, mostly plant-based diet, or in a quality supplement with higher bioavailability (i.e., liposomal delivery or other novel delivery systems).

- **Quercetin** – topical application helps reduce skin inflammation caused by *P. acnes*.[151]
- **Resveratrol** – oral administration has antioxidant and antiglycation activity which helps reduce the production of AGEs.[152] Topical administration has a skin lightening effect.[153]
- **Coenzyme Q_{10}** – topical administration in combination with strawberry polyphenols and SPF protects skin cells against UVA damage.[154] Topical CoQ_{10} along with vitamin E may also help with damage caused by UVB radiation.[155]
- **Curcumin** – topical and oral administration helps in the treatment of psoriasis, atopic dermatitis, and other inflammatory skin conditions by suppressing inflammation.[156] Topicals frequently contain other botanicals along with curcumin.
- **Capsaicin** – topical creams, and gels are quite effective in the elimination of skin inflammation, psoriasis, atopic dermatitis, and shingles, as well as the pain and itch experienced with these conditions.[157] Look for supplements with the branded ingredient Capsiatra®. It provides the benefits of capsaicin without the pungency.

- **Alpha Lipoic Acid** – the preferred administration has been oral or injection, but recently-developed topical applications have improved skin permeability and resulted in epidermal thickening and reduced skin pigmentation.[158]
- **N-Acetylcysteine** – oral supplementation has proved valuable for some patients suffering with pathological grooming disorders, such as skin picking, hair pulling, or nail biting who do not respond to pharmacologic or psychological treatment.[159]

Essential Fatty Acids

In Chapter 2, I discussed the importance of essential fatty acids (EFAs)—the omega-3s and omega-6s—and their contribution to healthy-looking, non-dry, non-flaky skin. Since the body cannot manufacture EFAs, we must get them from foods or supplements.

For non-vegans, krill oil and fish oil are excellent choices. Krill oil is somewhat better than fish oil because of its high phospholipid content which helps the body absorb it more easily; the amount of krill oil needed is about one-third less than fish oil. Vegetarians can benefit from plant-based EFA supplements, too. These include flaxseed oil, algae oil, and perilla oil (from the *perilla frutescent* plant). Although available in liquid form, capsules or softgels are generally more palatable and more convenient to take. I routinely take a product from Enzymedica called AquaBiome™ Fish Oil + Meriva Curcumin. The specialized, more absorbable type of curcumin provides extra help in combatting inflammation. There is, however, a precaution if you supplement with very high doses of omega-3s; a small amount of research suggests that this may cause atrial fibrillation.[160] Discuss this with your doctor, especially if you have heart issues or a family history.

Hyaluronic Acid

Hyaluronic acid (HA) is perhaps best known for its joint lubrication ability (i.e., moisture in the synovial fluid), but it also helps skin retain moisture. The ability for the skin to stay hydrated not only prevents irritation but also helps protect against damaging UV exposure. Essentially, HA "plumps" up the skin so minor flaws are less noticeable. The body's natural HA reserves diminish over time, which becomes increasingly evident as the skin's own hyaluronic acid-producing cells begin to taper off. When we look in the mirror, we see noticeable fine lines, uneven tone and texture, dullness, and later on…distinct wrinkles.

Hyaluronic acid is typically thought of as a topical product, and yes, incorporating a HA serum into your antiaging skincare regime is recommended. (See PART III: What Topicals Should I Apply?) Use of oral HA as a skin-health supplement is gaining in popularity, due in part to new research focusing on the "beauty from within" concept. Manufacturers have been able to make the HA molecules smaller so as to increase absorption in the GI tract and increase effectiveness in both skin and joint tissue.

Most hyaluronic acid supplements are derived from the combs of roosters (coxcomb), the red colored flesh that protrudes from a rooster's head. This type of HA is similar to our natural HA, but because it's sourced from an animal, nutraceutical use is not acceptable to vegans and strict vegetarians. A non-animal-based HA is produced by bacterial fermentation. This is typically used in topical skincare products. A few companies use a combination of the two to create their powdered HA, so be sure to read product labels if you have specific dietary preferences.

Collagen Peptides

Collagen peptides are structural proteins which make up the connective tissues within the human body—bones, joints, skin, hair, and fingernails. There are five types of collagen (Types I, II, III, V, X); Type I comprises 90% of the body's collagen and provides structural benefits to the tissues I just mentioned. With respect to skin, Types I and III are recommended because they help improve the structure of the skin's surface and increase elasticity. This can help promote firmer, smoother skin and fewer wrinkles. The goal is to help replace the natural collagen loss that happens with normal aging.

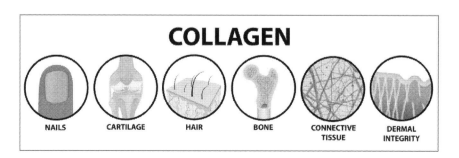

Different Types of Collagen	**TYPE I** • Comprises 90% of hair, skin, nails, organs, bones, and ligaments • Supports healthy, youthful skin	**TYPE II** • Helps build cartilage and maintains gut lining • Supports joint and digestive health • Promotes immune function
	TYPE III • Supports skin and bone health • Encourages arterial wall & cardiovascular health	**TYPE V/X** • Type V forms cell membranes and placenta tissue • Type X helps form bones

As a dietary supplement, collagen peptides contain most of the essential amino acids necessary for protein formation, with the three most prevalent being glycine, hydroxyproline, and proline. These proteins are commonly sourced from non-plant-based species, including marine (fish scales and skin), bovine (cow bones and skin), porcine (pig bones and skin), or poultry (chicken bones). The collagen is broken down, or hydrolyzed, into peptides that are easy to mix in liquids and are easily digestible in the GI tract. You'll often see the term "hydrolyzed" on these products. By comparison, collagen from bone broth, such as beef or chicken, is not hydrolyzed and not as easily digested.

The two most widely recommended collagen peptide supplements for skin health and beauty are marine and bovine-sourced. These collagen peptides are most definitely not for vegans or vegetarians. Dietary choices based on religious beliefs or preferred eating styles may necessitate supplements with marine or bovine (Kosher, Halal), or simply marine (pescatarian) sources. Other considerations include refining your choices—products derived from grass-fed, pasture-raised cattle (Types I and III collagen) or sustainably-raised fish (Type I collagen).

Once you've decided which source of collagen peptide is right for you, be sure to select one that doesn't add sugars or artificial sweeteners—there's no reason to promote further glycation in your existing collagen. Remember: You're trying to exit the skin collagen-glycation cycle. Plain collagen peptides have very little taste, and when they are added to a smoothie, mixed in a green drink, or dissolved into tea or coffee, the taste is unnoticeable (for most people).

There continues to be a fair amount of skepticism on the part of dermatologists as to whether oral collagen peptides do much for the skin. The amino acids in collagen are present in many foods, like wild salmon, egg yolks, and meats. In the absence of an enzyme deficiency, the body is quite adept at absorbing amino acids from all sources. I encourage people to consider collagen as an ingredient in skin health formulations in which other more well-documented ingredients such as antioxidants, vitamins, and minerals are providing most of the benefit.

Mushrooms

Most people have pretty strong feelings about edible fungi—either you like mushrooms, or you don't. And unless you're a mycologist (a biologist who specializes in fungi), you probably don't equate a brown fungus with beauty, further proving the old adage that beauty is truly in the eye of the beholder. In recent years, however, mushrooms—and mushroom supplements specifically—have gained in popularity as nutritional powerhouses offering immune support, cognitive support, and sleep support, alongside benefits for fitness and recovery, weight management, stress reduction, and of course, beauty. Since we're just talking beauty, I'll limit this section to the effects on skin. (Feel free to investigate the other areas on your own. You just might become a mushroom lover after all.)

The primary active ingredients in "medicinal mushrooms" are antioxidants and beta glucans, a type of soluble fiber. Antioxidants include glutathione, ergothioneine, polyphenols, flavonoids, and super oxidase dismutase (SOD). Beta glucans support gut health and skin health in multiple ways, with one very important function—serving as a prebiotic for the gut microbiome. So, even if you don't love mushrooms, the beneficial microbes in your gut do.

Benefits of Mushrooms on Skin Health[161,162]
- Improve digestion and protect the GI tract
- Modulate inflammation
- Neutralize free radicals
- Neutralize the damaging effects of stress
- Increase blood flow to the skin
- Down-regulate histamine-mediated allergic responses

Different mushroom species have different functions. Of the 3,283 edible species, we've really only begun to scratch the surface in terms of their applications outside of mere food. Lion's Mane (*Hericium erinaceus*) and Shiitake (*Lentinula edodes)* are known for soothing the GI tract, improving digestion, and increasing the good gut bacteria.[163,164] Chaga *(Inonotus obliquus)* has been shown to scavenge free radicals, thereby preventing UV-damaged skin cells from dying prematurely.[165] My favorite brand is Om Mushroom Superfood® (ommushrooms.com) which offers both capsules and powders for mixing into beverages. Their mushrooms are organic, non-GMO, and grown in the United States.

Ceramides

Ceramides (lipids) are key to the skin's barrier function, yet as the skin ages, the amount of natural ceramides contained in the outermost layer of the skin surface begins to wane. In turn, this increases the amount of water (moisture) which is lost. Depending on whether you can re-hydrate adequately or not, your skin can become dry and more susceptible to redness, irritation, and peeling. People who have eczema or rosacea tend to have lower-than-normal levels of ceramides. Eating a healthy diet with good fats from plant sources, ceramide-rich foods (See chapter 3 for a list.), and plenty of water is beneficial. Of course, if you live in an arid climate, dry skin is more of an issue, and you may want to consider a ceramide supplement.

Ceramide supplements can come from natural sources, such as wheat, rice, and sweet potatoes, or they can be manufactured (synthetic). If you normally exclude wheat from your diet, be sure to check the labels. There hasn't been a lot of clinical research on the effectiveness of oral ceramides, but the interest is quite high, as is for many ingestible skincare products. One such product that was approved by Health Canada (similar to our FDA) in 2018 is Myoceram. These rice-derived ceramides help replenish the lost ceramides so the skin can maintain its water-holding capacity. A clinical trial of the granular powder Myoceram found less water loss and improved skin conditions on the cheek, elbow, neck, and upper back after 4 weeks of use, and on the top surface of the foot after 8 weeks of use.[166]

Myoceram has been used for many years in Japan and other Asian countries, and more recently has come to North American markets. Myoceram and similar products are typically included as one of several ingredients in an ingestible skincare product.

Probiotics

As I've mentioned multiple times throughout *FYSR*, gut health is paramount to skin health. Thus, taking a quality probiotic supplement can help balance the gut microbiome and, in turn, encourage healthy, beautiful-looking skin. My personal recommendations are in Chapter 4: How Your Gut-Brain-Skin are All Connected.

Nitric Oxide Supplements

Nitric oxide is a compound produced naturally in the body and is recognized by every cell. It causes blood vessels to dilate, basically relaxing the smooth muscle around the small and large arteries and allowing them to relax. This increases blood flow and provides more oxygen to the body's tissues. If skin cells don't get enough blood blow and oxygen, they don't perform at their best.

According to molecular and physiology expert Nathan Bryan, PhD, it's important to remember that "Nitric oxide is a gas that diffuses throughout the body. We can even detect nitric oxide coming off the skin," which is actually a good thing. Nitric oxide supplements are typically formulated from a combination of beets and greens. The salivary glands and oral bacteria play an essential role in converting the nitrate and nitrite in plants to nitric oxide in the human body.

Two great supplements to boost your nitric oxide are Neo40®, a dissolvable oral tablet from HumanN (humann.com), and Berkeley Life Nitric Oxide Support (berkeleylife.com), available as a capsule. The Berkeley Life product features a healthy dose of the amino acid L-arginine blended with additional ingredients such as beetroot, L-citrulline, pine bark, and fenugreek. Both companies also make test strips you can put in your mouth to get a read out on your nitric oxide levels. A few other products I recommend for vascular health are Resync Recovery Blend (resyncproducts.com), a plant-based nitric oxide booster and AG1™ from Athletic Greens® (athleticgreens.com), a green drink powder with 75 whole-food sourced nutrients.

Glutathione

This antioxidant, also known by its acronym (GSH), is produced by the liver from three amino acids—glycine, cysteine, and glutamic acid. Aside from its free radical-squelching activity, glutathione plays a role in tissue building and repair which supports skin health. Unfortunately, poor nutrition (the SAD), toxin exposure, and too much inflammation all deplete glutathione. The big problem with glutathione supplementation is its poor oral absorption. Because of this, some in the medical community discount its effectiveness as a nutritional supplement. It has also been suggested that taking the glutathione precursors (glycine, cysteine, and glutamic acid) is more doable.

Glutathione is one of the most common ingredients added to IV drip nutrient therapy, most commonly as a "push" in a mixture of vitamins and minerals known as a Myer's cocktail. This mixture consists of magnesium, calcium, and vitamin C. Alan Gaby, MD, presented some of the early reports on the rationale for use of IV drips as therapy for a broad spectrum of diseases.[167] Glutathione is often used intravenously because of its generally poor oral absorption.

Given the powerful antioxidant benefits of GSH, some skincare formulators are creating topicals incorporating this molecule. A 10-week study of a topical GSH on Japanese women showed improvement in skin whitening and wrinkle reduction. Unfortunately, because glutathione is a sulfur-containing molecule, there is initially an egg smell upon application that gradually fades over time.[168]

> ### IV DRIPS: MY PERSPECTIVE
> Many functional medicine-oriented physicians offer IV nutrient treatment. It can be most helpful for people with significant GI absorption issues. I have personally used IV drips a few times, usually around the onset or tail end of an upper respiratory infection. I believe that the long haul (good nutrition and intelligent oral supplementation) is far superior to periodic blasts of megadoses of basic vitamins and minerals. Specific combinations of nutrients may play a role in helping with chronic diseases, but for skin beauty, I wouldn't place all my bets on getting IVs. Be advised that high doses of intravenous glutathione have been associated with side effects, such as rashes.[169]

Glutathione is the master detoxification supplement in the body and so I lean on it for general well-being. I'll often load up a bit before, during, and after travelling. In order to get better oral absorption, supplement manufacturers are delivering glutathione (and other nutrients) in liposomes, small nano-sized encapsulations of active ingredients. The liposome protects the nutrient from being destroyed by the stomach acid and allows better absorption from the intestines. My personal favorite liposomal glutathione supplement is from Quicksilver Scientific (quicksilverscientific.com). It comes in a convenient travel size pump that dispenses the liquid liposomal formulation.

NAD+

Nicotinamide adenine dinucleotide (NAD+) is a coenzyme that's produced naturally in every cell of the body and its primary purpose is to help power the mitochondria. It also plays a role in cellular repair that results from poor lifestyle (i.e., overeating, drinking alcohol, lack of exercise, insufficient sleep, psychological stress). The NAD+ building blocks are the vitamin B3s—niacin, nicotinamide, and nicotinamide riboside. These are found in B3-rich foods, including cow's milk, fish, green-colored vegetables, mushrooms, and yeast, as well as vitamin B3 supplements.

After the age of 40, NAD+ levels decrease by greater than 50%.[170] Low NAD+ is associated with mitochondrial inefficiency, or deficiency, depending how you look at it. The bottom line is that it affects aging—in a very big way. It's the degradation of cells, in this case, skin cells that make us look (and feel) old. To counter this negative effect, I routinely take Qualia Life (neurohacker.com) an NAD+ supplement that has shown significant improvement in selected biomarkers after both 5 days and 4 weeks. There is good science to support the more well-known Tru Niagen® (truniagen.com). It is a daily supplement from ChromaDex which increases NAD+ levels so skin cells can function properly.

Supplements Do Serve a Purpose

I'm an unabashed proponent of whole food eating to supply macro and micronutrients. I love shopping at my local farmers market (and growing a few fruits and vegetables of my own) for the most nutrient-dense, organic, and incredibly fresh foods. This doesn't always fit everyone's personal needs or lifestyle, so if you need a supplement(s), be sure to choose high-quality, reputable brands. Your body runs on the fuel you provide it, so make sure it's premium grade. The bottom line is that if a combination of whole foods and supplements can give you the great-looking, natural-looking, and healthy skin you desire—without expensive or risky cosmetic procedures—go for it! But, if you want a little extra insurance, are experiencing an acute or chronic condition, or have a genetic variant or take a drug which predisposes you to a deficiency, supplements can definitely make a difference.

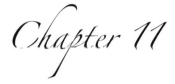

Chapter 11

HOW TO PERSONALIZE YOUR SUPPLEMENT REGIMEN

A Bit of Self-Disclosure

I am often asked the question, "Dr. Tager, what supplements do you take?" In this chapter I will offer a bit about my personal narrative. Keep in mind that what is right for me is not necessarily right for you. You may need to adjust your plan for skin conditions such as acne, eczema, or psoriasis. Or modify it based on gut health, genetics, environment, allergies; stage in life, or how much you are willing or able to spend on supplements. Also, not everyone reacts the same way to any given product, so if you notice issues—mainly GI problems—or have an allergy to any of the ingredients, then that supplement is not for you. You need a reason—ideally drawn from data—to take a given supplement.

I take this supplement because_____. (Fill in the reason.)

This is a chapter dedicated to filling in the blanks.

Get Your Base Needs Met

Summertime, sunny San Diego, eating from my garden and farmers markets, I will often skip taking a baseline vitamin and mineral supplement. When the weather turns cold, or I'm flying a lot, not getting enough sleep, or under/over exercising, I'll take a multivitamin mineral supplement, sometimes daily, sometimes every other day, to augment intelligent food choices.

There is a tendency on the part of manufacturers to overload multivitamin mineral supplements so they can claim their product is the strongest. It's not uncommon to see RDAs of 1,000% (10X) or even 2,000% (20X) for some nutrients. As you consider a basic daily vitamin/mineral supplement, you can opt to get as many essential vitamins, minerals, and possibly phytonutrients in one pill, powder, gummy, or liquid. Many people think of this as a health-insurance policy. The challenge comes in when you want to layer on additional skin health and beauty supplements; you'll just need to be careful not to exceed upper tolerable levels for some of the fat-soluble vitamins and/or minerals.

For those who want the convenience of one daily pill, I recommend taking a multiple vitamin/mineral formulation from any of the professional or consumer companies described in Chapter 8. My personal approach is to take a basic vitamin/mineral multivitamin with modest amounts of the essentials—say 2-4 times the RDA 200%-400%—and then select the other nutrients based upon my individual needs. You can determine your individual needs by addressing the following categories.

Supplements to Protect Your Skin from the Inside Out

The growth in this entire category of products has manufacturers scrambling to develop all-in-one formulas. Because many people have their preferred route of administration i.e., capsule, powder, or liquid, I've broken my recommendations into these three categories. Gummies are great, but there's only so much active ingredient you can cram into them. I routinely take the all-in-one supplements for each of the three categories, depending upon my mood, taste, and travel schedule.

Qualia Skin™ (neurohacker.com) is a capsule that contains a blend of minerals, bamboo, lycopene, buckthorn, and some excellent branded ingredients including Bionap's Red Orange Complex™ antioxidants, Pomanox™ pomegranate, and Hydropeach™ ceramides. I am a big fan of the branded Mediterranean antioxidants in Qualia Skin. Capsules are extremely convenient for traveling.

Regenacol™ Skin Inside® (sovereignlaboratories.com). A newer product with powdered bovine Colostrum-LD® as its base, it includes well recognized ingredients for gut and skin health including collagen, hyaluronic acid, zinc carnosine, Myoceram® ceramides, lycopene, and vitamin C. The product is flavored with monk fruit and tastes (to my taste buds) good when mixed in water. I often throw liposomal bovine colostrum into shakes, so now I use Skin Inside® instead. Some people need to go slowly with colostrum use because of initial digestive issues. In this case, you can start with half-servings and then gradually building up to the full amount.

Aethern® (aethern.com) A daily skin drink dispensed in individual shots, the formula contains bioactive collagen peptides, hyaluronic acid, astaxanthin, silicon, magnesium, zinc, beta-carotene, calcium, lutein, selenium, and a mixture of Mediterranean antioxidant polyphenols. Two highly regarded dermatologists, Jeffrey Dover, MD and Zoey Draelos, MD did the clinical studies that showed improvements in skin hydration, radiance, and firmness. When the product first came out some years ago, there were challenges with the taste. They've solved this issue and I actually look forward to my morning dose.

Skinade® (skinade.com) is a competitive liquid product featuring marine collagen and multiple active ingredients. Another liquid formulation comes from **Bend Beauty** (bendbeauty.com). I don't have any personal experience with these two products. Liquid formulations have to taste good in order for you to keep taking them. As we've learned from the chapter on nutrigenomics, our genes influence our taste perception, and what appeals to one person's palate may not appeal to another's.

Supplements to Support Your Blood Vessels

Arterial health is critical for skin beauty. Like the lining of the GI tract, the 60,000 miles of your blood vessels are lined by a very thin cellular layer, the epithelium. It is all too easy to damage this gateway into the body. High blood pressure, the oxidation of cholesterol, and toxins from oral bacteria all initiate inflammation. The result can be a thickening of the arterial wall, or worse yet, a clot that can block blood flow. When the small vessels of the skin are impacted, you lose that rosy glow of youth. As noted earlier, I lean heavily on omega-3 fatty acids, and routinely take either Neo40® which dissolves in my mouth, or Berkeley Life. I periodically add Arterosil® to my regimen. Arterosil® is a green seaweed-derived product that has been shown to promote a healthy glycocalx, the microscopic gel-like lining that naturally protects the endothelium of the arteries.

Supplements for Mitochondrial Energy Production

I'm a big believer in Co-Q10 and magnesium for mitochondrial energy support. The leading consumer brand of Co-Q10 is Qunol MegaCoQ10 Ubiquinol (qunol.com) which is available at an attractive price point. I personally rely on MitoQ®, influenced in large part by their clinical study showing significant improvement in blood pressure.[171] Another powerful mitochondrial enhancer is glutathione, and as I mentioned previously, my favorite formulation is Quicksilver Scientific's Liposomal Glutathione. It comes in a convenient spray. Because glutathione contains an amino acid with sulfur, there is a slight egg-taste to the liquid, which quickly goes away.

As I'm aging (*aren't we all?*), I find the need to maintain muscle mass in both my body and face. Preferring powders, I've long used aminoLIFE™ (amino-life.com), an amino acid-based supplement that has been shown to sustain lean muscle mass and muscle growth. It consists of a proprietary blend of high purity amino acids that do not contain fillers, toxins, or heavy metals, called Amino L40®.

Supplements that Help with Sleep

I've been pretty blessed with the ability to close my eyes and fall asleep anytime and anywhere. I think this is a holdover from medical training and residency, when you grabbed a few winks whenever you could. My wife of 37 years, however, has a tendency at night to perseverate on problems both real and imaginary, which cuts deeply into her sleep. (Hopefully, she won't read this far into the book.) We address this with magnesium (either bisglycinate or threonate) before bed, as well as combinations of melatonin, GABA (a naturally occurring neurotransmitter that signals the brain to calm down) and the amino acid L-theanine. These nutrients, in combination with good sleep hygiene (a dark and cool room, avoidance of blue light) plus grandparent duty—which renders her fairly exhausted—seem to do the trick.

There is a bit of trial and error in determining which sleep-promoting nutrients will work best for you. The popular adaptogen, ashwagandha, can be helpful, along with other botanicals such as chamomile, valerian root, and lavender to get to sleep. Some people utilize full-spectrum hemp extract. The few times I tried it—just to sample the effects—I had some weird dreams.

Pure Encapsulations (pureencapsulations.com) professional grade Best Rest Formula includes melatonin, GABA, L-theanine, valerian root, lemon balm, passionflower, chamomile, and hops. Many functional medicine physicians recommend NeuroCalm™, a product by Designs for Health.

For those who can fall asleep, but have trouble staying asleep, time-released melatonin may work better than regular melatonin. I recommend one or two tablets of Melatonin PR by Douglas Laboratories taken at bedtime. Another great supplement is LipoCalm from Quicksilver Scientific or Liposomal Zen (allergyresearchgroup.com). Both are liquids in an easy-to-spray bottle. These formulations can help you get back to sleep quickly and usually do not result in additional morning drowsiness.

For those with anxiety and/or depression, with trouble staying asleep, using 500 to 1000mg of tryptophan at bedtime can help keep serotonin levels stable to help you stay asleep.[172,173] For those who are super stressed out with high cortisol levels at night, taking supplements like ashwagandha, magnolia and phosphatidylserine (mentioned in Chapter 6) can help you sleep like a baby.

Neurohacker Collective® (neurohacker.com) took another approach to creating their Qualia Night Sleep Aid formulation. Rather than just focus on sleep, the scientists asked a more insightful question, "What nutrients do people need at night to recharge better for the next day?" The result was a formulation of 25 powerful ingredients including therapeutic mushrooms, herbs, roots, minerals and seeds. The product is designed to be taken 5 days on and 2 days off each week.

Supplements to Counter Drug-Nutrient Depletions

Almost half, 45.8% of Americans report using prescription drugs in the previous month, according to a 2015-2016 National Health and Nutrition Examination Survey.[174] Prescription drug use also increases as we grow older—from 18.0% of children under 12 to 85.0% of adults over 60. In the course of performing their intended functions, drugs can interact with the nutrients in foods (a drug-nutrient interaction, or DNI) and drugs can cause nutrient depletions (a drug-induced nutrient depletion, or DIND). The next chart describes many of the interactions. Always tell your prescribing physician what supplements you are taking, and always ask what nutrients may be affected by prescribed drugs.

COMMON DRUG-INDUCED NUTRIENT DEPLETIONS

MEDICATION	USE	EFFECT ON SPECIFIC NUTRIENTS
Proton Pump Inhibitors (PPIs)	Reduce stomach acid – heartburn, acid reflux, GERD, peptic ulcers	Inhibit the absorption of nutrients, such as B12, vitamin C, calcium, iron, magnesium
Statins	Lower cholesterol levels – help prevent cardiovascular disease	Inhibit the synthesis of nutrients, such as selenium, CoQ10, omega-3 fatty acids, fat soluble vitamins
Metformin	Lower blood glucose – type 2 diabetes, pre-diabetes	Alter the transport of nutrients, such as folate, B12
ACE Inhibitors	Lower blood pressure – hypertension	Increase or decrease the excretion of nutrients from the body, such as zinc
Antibiotics	Kill infectious bacteria – ear, lung, kidney, skin infections, acne, food poisoning	Inhibit the absorption of nutrients, such as vitamin K, folic acid, B vitamins
Estrogens	Restore/increase estrogen levels – hormone replacement therapy, oral birth control	Increase or decrease the metabolism of nutrients, such as B12, B6, folic acid, riboflavin, magnesium, zinc, tyrosine, vitamin C

> ## NUTRIENT-NUTRIENT INTERACTIONS
>
> Nutrients can interact with each other (a nutrient-nutrient interaction, or NNI), but that's not always a bad thing. Synergistic nutrient combinations enhance their functionality—the sum is sometimes greater than the parts. Synergistic combinations include vitamin D and calcium, vitamin D and magnesium, and vitamin C and iron. Antagonistic nutrient combinations, on the other hand, are responsible for a decrease in the absorption or activity of one of the two nutrients. Common NNIs with inhibitory impacts include iron and calcium, zinc and copper, B12 and folate, and fluoride and iodine.
>
> - Calcium inhibits iron absorption.
> - Zinc inhibits copper's absorption.
> - A B12 deficiency renders folic acid inactive.
> - Fluoride contributes to iodine deficiency.

Self-Care Tip: Given how many medications are out there, and all the possible interactions, you can always check your drug/nutrient interactions by using Mytavin.com. This compendium, originally developed by Jeff Gladd, MD, is being used both by professionals and consumers.

Supplements to Compensate for Genetic-Related Insufficiencies

If you have the opportunity to assess your nutrition-related SNPs, go for it. (Refer to the list of companies in Chapter 5.) In addition to learning I had a genetic risk variant that predisposed me to low vitamin D, I also learned that I would benefit from additional zinc, vitamin E, and choline. While I sometimes take liquid choline (Perque Choline Citrate™ perque.com), which is critical for nerve function, most of my choline comes from eating free-range chicken eggs (with those incredible orange yolks).

Supplements to Support Immunity

With the pandemic in mind, or hopefully in the rear-view mirror, nonetheless it seems that every supplement manufacturer has pivoted to noting that their product "supports immune health." I make certain my vitamin D levels are in the optimal range, that I'm consuming a good blend of antioxidants and specifically decent quantities of vitamin C (1,000-2,000 mg/day). Put another way, I'm not doing anything different from my normal routine which is already immune-supportive.

Supplements that Build the Microbiome

I really rely on fiber-rich prebiotics and fermented foods for my gut-skin health, and with the exception of SereneSkin™ (microbiomelabs.com) which contains a healthy blend of bacillus species, I don't usually take a supplemental probiotic. Some thoughts on selecting a probiotic:

- **The type of bacteria.** You would be well advised to note the distinctions that the professional supplement companies make in terms of blends of Lactobacilli such as *L. acidophilus, Bifidobacterium bifidum*, and different Bacillus species including *B. coagulans*, all of which have gut-skin benefits.
- **Acne.** In the last five years alone, more than 18,000 peer-reviewed studies on probiotics have been published, and many of these examined the role of specific bacteria strains on acne. The consensus is that mild to moderate acne can benefit from an oral probiotic supplement in addition to the standard treatment.[175] Some of the more noteworthy beneficial strains include *Staphylococcus epidermidis, Streptococcus salivarius, Lactococcus sp. HY449, Streptococcus thermophiles, Lactobacillus paracasei, Enterococcus faecalis*, and *Lactobacillus plantarum*.[176]
- **Photoaging.** UV-induced skin damage may be partially remedied by probiotics which improve the skin's barrier function (decreases moisture loss) and reduce oxidative stress in the skin (decreases inflammation). Bacterial strains advantageous to skin anti-aging include *Bifidobacterium breve, Lactobacillus plantarum* HY7714, *Lactobacillus rhamnosus* GG, *Lactobacillus casei, Lactobacillus johnsonii*, and *Lactobacillus johnsonii* NCC 533.[177]
- **Anti-Aging.** Healthy, "young" skin has a slightly acidic pH (4.2-5.6) which helps maintain moisture, but after age 70, pH rises significantly and becomes alkaline. This compromises the skin's barrier function, so consuming probiotics which produce acidic molecules (i.e., lactic acid) when they are metabolized is likely to return the skin's pH level to a "younger" level. Lactobacilli species are efficient lactic acid-producing bacteria and are found in many probiotic supplements.

- **The number of organisms.** As measured in colony-forming units (CFUs), there should be a minimum of 10-20 billion per serving.
- **Third-party certification.** Reputable organizations include Consumer Labs, US Pharmacopeia (USP), and NSF International.
- **Probiotic form.** Probiotics come in tablets, capsules, liquids, and powders, so choose based on which form is easiest for you to swallow. Probiotics are either shelf-stable or refrigerated. There is no specific benefit to refrigerated probiotics. The important thing is to use the probiotic before expiration date to ensure the maximum number of bacteria are still alive.
- **Professional grade.** As with other types of supplements such as fish oils, I believe you will have the assurances of safety, potency, and purity if you stick to the supplement companies recommended in *FYSR*.

Supplements to Help Regulate Insulin Resistance/Glycation

The big thing here is to cut out simple carbs and sugars. The power of dietary supplements pales in the face of the onslaught from spikes in blood sugar levels. Chromium, magnesium, and resveratrol have some benefits in carbohydrate metabolism and insulin sensitivity. Berberine is a plant molecule extracted from the plant *berberis*, and has been shown to increase insulin sensitivity and lower blood sugar. Most of the professional supplement companies make pure forms, including OrthoMolecular Products and Enzymedica.

Find the Timing That Works for You

By now you're probably wondering how to juggle all these recommendations. As a basic guideline, here's what I do: Since I often practice time-restricted eating—finishing dinner at 7-8 pm and not eating anything until 8-10 am the next morning—I usually take my all-in-one skin supplement (Qualia Skin or Aethern) around 10 am; alternatively, I take a scoop of Regenacol Skin Inside either with water or in a morning shake. I take my fat soluble or fat-loving supplements—vitamin D_3K2 combo, Enzymedica's AquaBiome + Meriva Curcumin, and my delta-tocotrienols—either with a fat-containing breakfast or dinner. If I'm going out to eat, I usually take DigestGold just prior to dinner. I will take my aminoLIFE, MitoQ and Qualia Life prior to or just after working out; sometimes I'll substitute ReSync or a greens drink. For much of the year, I rely on a multi-vitamin and make certain I'm getting 1,000mg-2,000mg of vitamin C each day. When I remember, right after dinner, I usually take a magnesium supplement (which ironically, should help me remember to take it more frequently).

Suffice it to say, at this point, you know way too much about me, my daily habits, and my approach to dietary supplements. I am not one who believes in going overboard. I am pretty good about adhering to this plan. I do notice a falloff in my energy, loss of a bit of glow in my skin, and some changes in body composition when I stray from this approach. This is my regimen and the way I fill in the blanks. How you fill in the blanks is up to you. I hope you've gained the information and framework to decide what's *right* for you.

Part Three: What Topicals Should I Apply?

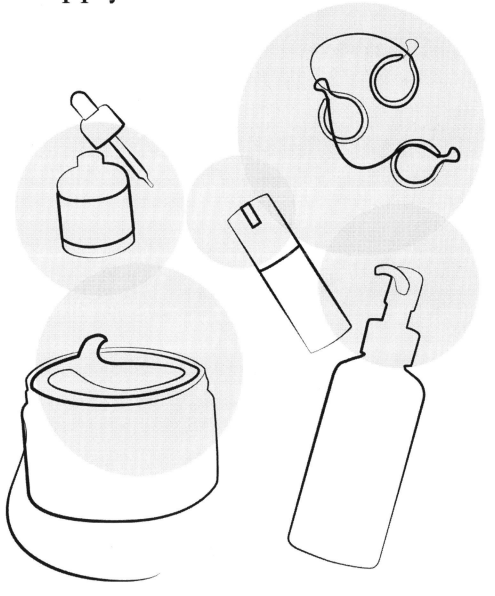

"I'm a big believer that if you focus on good skin care, you really won't need a lot of make-up."

Demi Moore

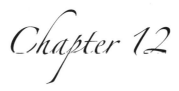

TOPICALS: WHAT ACTUALLY WORKS?

Get the Odds in Your Favor

I'm a firm believer in the Pareto Principle—the 80/20 rule—that says that, in a given list, 80% of the value or benefit comes from just 20% of the items. This is my philosophy when it comes to topicals. You'll get 80% of your skin beauty by shielding your sun from the skin with protective clothing, applying a mineral-based sunblock, drinking enough water, eating a nutrient-rich diet with intelligent supplementation, and applying a few topicals to hydrate, protect, and counter oxidative damage. All the professional "medical grade" companies, and many of the direct-to-consumer companies, have products that will fit the bill. Most have gone through rigorous product tests. (See below.) With more than 15,000 products on the market, the challenge is finding the ones that are right for you.

> ### PRODUCT TESTING
> The most reputable topical product companies do the following:
> - **Clinical testing for claim substantiation**. This allows the company to make certain claims, i.e., "85% of participants noticed improvement in wrinkles."
> - **48-hour irritancy study**. This determines if a product will irritate the skin.
> - **In-house consumer testing**. This usually involves 20-30 consumer test subjects who respond to questions about the product.
> - **The Repeat Insult Patch Test (RIPT)**. The RIPT identifies the likelihood that the product will cause skin rashes. This allows products to be labeled as "hypoallergenic."
> - **Testing for eye irritation**. This ensures that there will be no irritation should the product get into the eyes.
> - **Dermatologist formulated/dermatologist tested**. This refers to the level of involvement of skincare professionals with the product.

In the last decade, the difference between "medical grade" products and over-the-counter formulations has narrowed. The assumption is that medical grade products are stronger and more potent than "regular" skincare products. This is possible, but the reality is that any product can be too harsh for your skin. The significant difference is that the medical-grade products are often formulated by leading dermatologists, subjected to rigorous testing, made available in cosmetic practices, and most importantly, have published studies to support their efficacy. There are also prescription topicals which have gone through the FDA approval process and are only available from a physician.

Back to Pareto and the other 20%. This is where philosophy, science, and personal preference converge. Topicals fall into a few major categories. There are those that are specifically derived from plant sources and are marketed as more "natural." There are topicals that have the scientific molecule shown to be effective in the laboratory, or in a small clinical study to confer benefits for skin beauty. These ingredients are often hyped as the latest and greatest. All too often, they develop a fanbase for a while, then people go on to the next latest and greatest.

What Category of Topicals Stand the Test of Time?

In keeping with the personalized nature of *FYSR*, and the promise of helping you determine what to apply to your skin, here is my decision-tree, informed to a large degree by discussions with my favorite dermatologists. I asked them point blank how they go about assessing patient's topical needs, which categories of products are essential and worth the investment, and which should only be used in selected cases. As we progress through this chapter, you'll be hearing from some of the nation's top dermatologists including (alphabetically):

- Glynis Ablon, MD (abloninstitute.com)
- Shino Bay Aguilera, DO (shinobayderm.com)
- Sonia Badreshia-Bansal, MD (elitemdspa.com)
- Apple Bodemer, MD (dermatology.wisc.edu/staff/bodemer-apple)
- Suneel Chilukuri, MD (refreshdermatology.com)
- Doris Day, MD (dorisdaymd.com)
- Heidi Waldorf, MD (waldorfderm.com)

Take the Professional Route

While topicals can be found everywhere, what is much more precious is professional guidance. Even if you eventually choose to buy the recommended skincare products elsewhere, nothing replaces professional advice, including a thorough skin analysis (along with an annual check of your skin lesions). Many professionals are opting to create their own online formularies of the topicals they prefer. When you use these services for ordering your topicals, your physician can track which products you are using and, if necessary, easily make other recommendations if the products aren't suiting you.

Keep it Simple and Clean

Universally, leading dermatologists share the philosophy that "less is more." Most professionals personally use and recommend just a few select products to be applied on a daily basis. Contrast this with the statistic that the average woman uses an average of 16 facial care or cosmetics products a day. This amounts to $200,000-$300,000 in a lifetime (or an estimated $250 per month).[178] Compounding this is a report from the Environmental Working Group, noting that in a typical day, the average woman applies products containing 168 different chemicals to her skin.[179] In general, avoid products that contain potential skin irritants such as parabens, synthetic fragrances, mineral oil, sulfate detergents, urea, or potentially carcinogenic substances phthalates and ethanolamines DEA or TEA.

While we're on the subject of cleanliness, you're best advised to use a gentle pH-balanced cleanser that protects the natural acid mantle of the skin, particularly if you are acne-prone. The acidic pH allows the good bacteria on your skin to flourish and discourages a takeover by the bad bugs. Dr. Bodemer notes that, "Anything that's foaming up in your hands is going to be really harsh on your skin. It's going to strip a lot of oil away from your skin. Along with the antibacterial soaps, when we strip that oil away too aggressively, we're telling the oil glands, 'You need to make more oil. You're not keeping up; we need more protection.' And so, the oil glands go into overdrive and that's where a vicious cycle starts." Dr. Ablon shares Bodemer's concerns and encourages her patients to use cleansing wipes as one way to avoid transferring foreign substances to the face.

The 80%: Your Foundation for Skin Health & Beauty

Adhering to the keep-it-simple principle, professionals divide the must-have products into four basic categories:

1. Sunblock
2. Barrier Protection
3. Retinoids
4. Antioxidants and/or Peptides

1. SUNBLOCK

While sunscreen is a loose term that can describe physical or chemical protection, sunblock is always used to describe physical UV protection. By shielding the skin from these harmful rays, you can prevent premature aging (loss of elasticity & wrinkling), tanning, and sunburns, as well as lower the risk of skin cancer.

All sun protection is graded according to the acronym SPF which stands for Sun Protection Factor. The Food and Drug Administration defines SPF as "a measure of how much solar energy (UV radiation) is required to produce sunburn on protected skin (i.e., in the presence of sunscreen) relative to the amount of solar energy required to produce sunburn on unprotected skin."[180] It's important to remember that SPF is unrelated to the actual time you spend in the sun before burning. So, yes, as the SPF number increases, sunburn protection also increases, but it also depends on the time of day, geographic location, clouds versus full sun, your skin type, how frequently you apply the sunblock, the extent to which you perspire, whether you immerse yourself in water, and whether you apply it sparingly (not good) or liberally (the way to go).

The universal recommendation of "my" dermatologists is to select a mineral sunblock, either with zinc and/or titanium oxide. Look for an SPF of around 30 or more. If you are participating in outdoor sports, consider an SPF of 50 or more. In addition to avobenzone and other chemicals being harmful for the coral reefs and outlawed in some ocean-facing states and territories, you don't need to add another chemical to your skin if you can avoid it. So, skip the chemical blocks.

The challenge with many of the physical blockers is they can be chalky. According to Dr. Badreshia-Bansal, for skin of color this often results in an ashen or dry look. Fortunately, many manufacturers are making ultra-sheer products, including Dr. Badreshia-Bansal who offers patients her BB

Primer Broad Spectrum SPF 50+ with zinc oxide and green tea (elitemdspa.com).

The minerals in these sheer preparations have been micronized or nano-sized—basically ground into very small particles. I've long been a fan of EltaMD®'s suite of sunblocks (eltamd.com) which go on smooth and are available in a number of formulations both tinted and non-tinted. In general, tinted formulas offer a small degree of extra protection and are often recommended for those with hyperpigmentation conditions such as melasma.

Dr. Waldorf notes that her patients will use sunblock only if they like the feel of it. Accordingly, she often recommends skinbetter science®'s sunbetter SHEER SPF 56 Sunscreen Stick with Titanium Dioxide 5.0% and Zinc Oxide 10.0% (sunbetter.com). She has found that the product is well-accepted by the men in her practice, as well as women. For those patients who prefer a powder that can be easily incorporated into a make-up regimen, she recommends ColorScience® (colorscience.com) all mineral Sunforgettable® Total Protection™ Brush-On Shield products available in a variety of SPFs. Dr. Ablon is partial to Revision Skincare's Intellishade® Clear-Clear. In addition to sunblock, it contains a blend of peptides and antioxidants. (Discussed in detail later.)

Some manufacturers are also adding DNA repair enzymes to their sunblocks. These bacterial-produced enzymes recognize and correct physical damage done to DNA by radiation, UV light, or reactive oxygen species (ROS). Proponents of these enzymes note that they penetrate the skin where they slow the progression of damage and reduce some of the effects of photoaging, as well as reduce the risk of certain skin cancers in high-risk patients.[181] Other researchers point to the need for more randomized controlled studies to show that sunscreens with DNA repair are more effective than conventional sunscreens.[182] Dr. Waldorf recommends ISDIN Eryfotona Actinica™ based upon the feel of the product as well as the DNA repair enzymes. Dr. Chilukuri similarly recommends ISDIN Eryfotona, especially to any person who has had a skin cancer.

Regardless of which sunblock product you elect to use, remember to use it every time you are outdoors (including driving in your car). And don't forget, the best protection is afforded by sun-protective clothing. Try to apply the sunblock 20 minutes before significant sun exposure.

2. BARRIER PROTECTION

Great looking skin is properly hydrated skin where water is not evaporating through epidermis cracks. Researchers most often assess the critical importance of the skin barrier, by measuring transepidermal water loss (TEWL). The goal of any barrier protection product is to reduce TEWL. The skin barrier is also vital as one of the first lines of defense for the immune system. Specialized cells called dendritic cells lie in the dermis and send their tentacle-like projections up into the epidermis to sense the presence of potentially harmful organisms. If they detect foreign substances, dendritic cells jumpstart the inflammatory cascade.

The purpose of moisturizers is to both hydrate and protect the skin. Lighter moisturizers tend to have more water in them and will offer less barrier protection. Heavier moisturizers will shield the skin more effectively from water loss (best applied at night). Serums offer very little barrier protection, so if you are going to use them, particularly at night, you'll want to layer a moisturizer over them.

There's a great deal of personal preference involved when it comes to moisturizers. Smell, feel, thickness, ease of spread, the degree of stickiness, and silkiness all come into play. Moisturizers also differ as to the presence and concentration of active ingredients such as antioxidants or peptides.

My personal approach as a simple guy is to use a light moisturizer during the day underneath my SPF, my preferences being Cetaphil® (cetaphil.com), CeraVE® (cerave.com), Epionce® (epionce.com), Spadr® (thespadr.com), or Vanicream™ (vanicream.com). At nighttime, I will usually go over to my wife's side of the bathroom and grab some of her heavier creams—the current ones being Estee Lauder Revitalizing Supreme+ (esteelauder.com) or AlphaScience's Ultra Firm (alphascience.com). I'll apply my retinol, or antioxidants/peptides beforehand. If retinoids irritate your skin, consider applying them after the moisturizer.

According to Dr. Waldorf, an effective moisturizer contains both humectants and emollients to retain water. You can think of humectants as little sponges, pulling water into the skin. Naturally occurring humectants are hyaluronic acid, glycerin, and even collagen. The emollients, on the other hand, are like little tarps: they cover the skin with a protective film to trap in water.

Although not universally recommended, Dr. Waldorf is in favor of dimethicone for its ability to impart a silky feeling with some slip to it. As a dermatologist, she washes her hands multiple times each day and relies on topical Replenix® (replenix.com) hand lotion, noting "It has glycerin and dimethicone; basically, dimethicone acts to seal in the skin and it make it silky, while the glycerin is holding in the moisture."

Manufacturers have been able to create smaller molecules of hyaluronic acid which can be an excellent humectant. Applying these as a serum can help boost hydration. There are multiple brands available at modest price points, with many combining antioxidant ingredients.

Dr. Shino Bay Aguilera's most recommended hyaluronic acid brand is HA Intensifier Serum from SkinCeuticals. It contains three different types of hyaluronic acid, proxylane (a glycoprotein that stimulates the GAGs in the extracellular matrix), and botanicals including licorice root extract and purple rice. The formulation supports the body's natural production of hyaluronic acid leading to significant improvement in skin plumpness, and reduction of lines, wrinkles, and folds.

Enhancing the Natural Skin Barrier

The quantity of natural ceramides in the outermost layers of the epidermis begins decreasing in the third and fourth decades of life—rather significantly, perhaps as great as 40% and 60% loss, respectively.[183] As such, you probably noticed that your skin became drier in your 30s and 40s. Unfortunately, ceramide and lipid loss continue as you age and without intervention, it's a downward spiral. The skin continues to lose its ability to retain moisture, the skin's barrier function is compromised, and the skin's surface pH increases—all signs of aging.[184]

Ceramides take on increasing importance for people who are experiencing irritation from topicals that accelerate skin turnover and exfoliation. These include retinoids, alpha hydroxy acids (AHAs) and polyhydrox acids (PHAs). Ceramides are also important to use both pre- and post-laser procedures. Fearing an increased risk of infection, many dermatologists will not perform skin resurfacing procedures on patients whose skin barrier function is compromised. They will perform the procedure after weeks of pre-laser topical treatment has healed the skin barrier. My go-to formulation for many years has been SkinMedica® TNS Ceramide Treatment Cream™ (skinmedica.com), which includes the TNS growth factors, peptides, and ceramides together in a reasonably affordable product.

Responding to many of her patient's price concerns, Dr. Bodemer will often steer people to Curél® (curel.com), Vanicream™, or Cetaphil® ceramide products. For patients who prefer more botanical products to soothe irritated skin, she will also recommend topicals by Avalon Organics® (avalonorganics.com), Weleda® Skin Food (weleda.com), and products by QET (qetbotanicals.com) which are based on infused oils. Another barrier-protective lipid ingredient to look for is squalane (not squalene). Originally sourced from the liver of sharks, it is now commonly obtained from olive oil, rice, and sugar cane and works as a moisturizing agent.

3. RETINOIDS

The anti-acne, anti-aging Retin-A® gel is probably the first product that comes to mind when you hear "retin"-something-or-other. As one of many topical retinoids, it's used by dermatologists to treat common inflammatory skin conditions, such as acne, as well as conditions related to slow skin cell turnover, such as psoriasis.

Dr. Chilukuri explains why and how retinoids are effective with acne. "On its own accord, the skin will turn over every 28 to 32 days. One of the causes of acne is that the skin clumps together, and as a result of clumping, even though we've produced the same amount of oil on a regular basis, we're not able to exfoliate that skin. So, with acne, we're seeing somewhere between 32 and 36 and sometimes 38 days for skin turnover. By using a topical retinoid, we can get the skin to turn over every seven days. That to me is a home run."

Because of this ability to dramatically ramp up skin cell turnover, most dermatologists consider retinoids as their number one treatment for anti-aging. Retinoids combat fine skin lines and wrinkles and stimulate collagen production. It takes about 12 weeks of consistent use to see significant results from treatment, whether the goal is acne improvement or wrinkle repair.

All Retinoids are Not the Same

Retinoids belong to a group of "vitamers" of vitamin A; vitamers are compounds that have similar chemical structure and function to that of a specific vitamin—in this case, vitamin A.

While some people use the terms retinoid and retinol interchangeably, it's important to note the differences. Retinoids are the overarching term used to describe all the different types of vitamin A derivatives.

The main difference between a retinol and a retinoid involves the strength of the ingredient. Retinols don't have as great a concentration of the active ingredient as retinoids. They are gentler on the skin, and it takes longer to see their effects. Retinols are available over-the-counter in various skin care products, while the most powerful retinoids are only available by prescription.

MEDICATION	AVAILABILITY & USE	PROPERTIES & BRAND NAMES
Retinyl Palmitate	OTC (anti-aging)	weakest retinoid; well-tolerated with low irritation; for sensitive or dry skin types
Retinol	OTC (anti-aging)	moderate strength retinoid; well-tolerated with mild irritation; for normal skin types
Retinaldehyde	OTC	increased strength and mild to moderate irritation; for normal skin types
Adapalene	OTC (anti-aging, acne)	strongest OTC retinoid which can also treat acne; for oily or acne-prone skin types
Tretinoin	Prescription (acne)	Retin-A®, Retin-A Micro®, Renova®, Tretin-X®, and Ziana®
Tazarotene	Prescription (psoriasis, acne scarring)	severe acne, and acne scars; Tazorac®

During the first couple weeks of using a retinoid product, people typically experience dry, flaky, and irritated skin, with an acne breakout not uncommon. This is simply an adjustment period as the skin responds to the retinoids and the faster rate of skin cell turnover. Retinoids can also make the skin more sensitive to the sun, so be sure to moderate your sun exposure and/or wear a cream with SPF 40+. You'll want to choose your over-the-counter (OTC) products based on your general skin type (dry, normal, or oily) and apply at night before going to bed, along with a moisturizer. If you require a prescription product, follow your dermatologist's instructions for best results.

Of all the dermatologists I consulted, none was more strident about retinoid use than Dr. Chilukuri, who declared that if he were ever stranded on a desert island, he would still want his retinoids with him. Dr. Chilukuri recommends PCA Skin® products (pcaskin.com) and points to the advantages of omnisome technology in PCA Skin's Retinol Treatment for Sensitive Skin 0.1% Retinol. The omnisome delivery technology encapsulates the unstable retinol molecule and allows for a slow release over ten hours. According to Dr. Chilukuri, this reduces the likelihood of irritation. For patients who still have difficulty with retinols, and desire the same effect, he recommends Isdin's Melatonik™ (isdin.com). The active skin turn-over accelerator ingredient is bakuchiol, an oil harvested from the native Indian plant babchi. Melatonik™ combines bakuchiol with vitamin C and melatonin for optimal results.

Dr. Shino Bay Aguilera's favorite retinol is prescription strength ReFissa® 0.05%. This is a tretinoin with an emollient cream base to improve tolerability. For those who want a non-Rx product, he recommends AlphaRet® by skinbetter science®. He has found it to produce good results with excellent tolerability.

I've personally had a hard time getting into the retinol habit. I have thin skin that is easily irritated. Every time I talk to my dermatology colleagues, especially Dr. Chilukuri, he reminds me that by using retinoids, I can get my skin to turn over in seven days. So, I start up again. I know that using retinoids (retinols for me) is especially important in the winter and fall months when my skin is already going to be dry. Here's the advice I've been given on how to make retinoids a habit:

- Apply a pea-sized amount and only at night.
- Moisturize like crazy. Go heavy at night.
- Always wear sun protection.
- Begin very gradually. Maybe one to three times a week, then move up slowly as tolerated.
- Have patience and stick with it. It will take several months to see results.

> **TRETINOIN IS NOT ISOTRETINOIN**
>
> Isotretinoin is another retinoid, available only by prescription. It is an oral drug available only for severe acne. Until 2009, it was only available by the brand name Accutane; now there are generic isotretinoins. Physicians who prescribe isotretinoin do it only for a finite period of time. The drug can't be used by people who are pregnant because it causes severe birth defects, as well as increases the risk of miscarriage and premature birth. All women of reproductive age who want to take isotretinoin must register with a program called iPledge in which they affirm they understand the risks and will avoid pregnancy.

4. ANTIOXIDANTS

The Gem that is Vitamin C

It's been just over twenty years since Duke professor of dermatology, Sheldon Pinnell, MD, published his work on the topical absorption of vitamin C. This small molecule remains the topical antioxidant standard to which all other antioxidants are measured. In addition to countering ROS, vitamin C strengthens collagen, and brightens the skin.[185]

Vitamin C is also the poster child for explaining the synergy of skin beauty inside and outside. When nutrients enter the bloodstream and make their way to the skin, their landing place is the dermis, the layer of the skin just beneath the epidermis. In addition to being home to the major nerves, blood vessels, sweat glands, and hair follicles, the space between these structures, the extracellular matrix (ECM) is equally important. It is where collagen, elastin, and a type of sugar-protein molecule known by the imposing name glycosaminoglycans reside. Skin professionals abbreviate glycosaminoglycans as "GAGs." The substances in the ECM are responsible for providing fullness and suppleness to the skin. When you are taking in minerals, vitamins, antioxidants, and other nutrients by mouth, they wind up in the dermis (where the action is).

The epidermis lacks the blood vessels that normally deliver nutrients to cells. In order for the ingested nutrients to reach the epidermis, they must diffuse from the dermis. Without blood flow, it's more difficult for the dietary nutrients to reach the cells in the outermost layers of the epidermis.

Topical delivery has always been thought of as an attractive way to get nutrients into the dermis. This isn't all that easy. The cells of the epidermis are packed tightly together, in essence, shielding the more metabolically active dermis. While some electrically charged and fat-soluble molecules can pass through many of the outer epidermal layers, most of the molecules applied to the skin won't make it to the dermis.[186] I'm sorry to break this to you, but the vast majority of topical products on the market today that claim to affect collagen and elastin, feature ingredients that are not reaching the dermis. They have no major effect on the skin beyond moisturization.

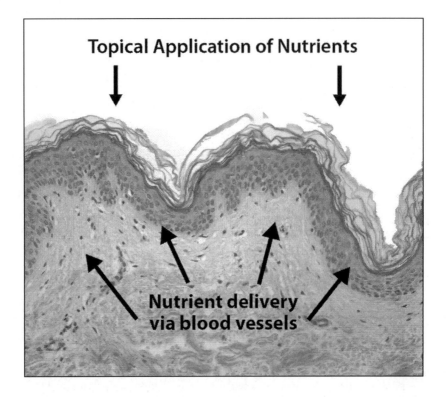

Vitamin C, by virtue of its molecular size and configuration, *does* penetrate the epidermis and reach the dermis where it can affect collagen, elastin, and the GAGs. This was the brilliance of Pernell's work. This realization led to the founding of SkinCeuticals (skinceuticals.com), the company behind CE Ferulic® the flagship product combining three powerful antioxidants: 15% L-ascorbic acid with vitamin E (as alpha tocopherol) and ferulic acid in a synergistic serum.

Not All Vitamin C is the Same

There are a half-dozen forms of vitamin C present in today's topical products. The most well-known and well-researched form is the L-ascorbic acid that is in the SkinCeuticals product. The concentration varies depending upon the manufacturer ranging from 10%-20%. The natural acidic pH of L-ascorbic acid will usually result in a product with a pH of less than 4. This works well for normal and oily skin types but can be irritating to sensitive skin.

Ascorbic acid is water-soluble and breaks down (oxidizes) when exposed to light and air. This inactivates the vitamin C. To keep the ingredients stable, ascorbic acid serums should be packaged in dark, opaque, glass droppers and kept out of the sun.

There are a number of other forms of vitamin C commonly used in skincare preparations, in large part because of their increased stability. These derivatives are helpful for people who can't tolerate ascorbic acid because of skin sensitivity. To be effective, most of these forms of vitamin C must be converted to ascorbic acid by the skin. This intermediate step renders them less potent. These derivatives include:

- Sodium ascorbyl phosphate
- Magnesium ascorbyl phosphate
- Sodium ascorbate
- Calcium ascorbate (Ester-C®)
- Ascorbyl palmitate
- Tetrahexyldecyl ascorbate

Vitamin C: Strength & Synergy

If your skin tolerates L-ascorbic acid serum, go for it. You'll be getting the gold standard. If the CE Ferulic® price point is too steep, a stepdown in price could be AlphaScience's Tannic CF serum (alphascience.com). It features 8% L-ascorbic acid along with phytic, and tannic acid obtained from sequoia bark.

You can also be on the lookout for synergistic ingredients. Vitamin C is more effective in the presence of vitamin E, as well as other antioxidants. SkinMedica's Vitamin C + E Complex (skinmedica.com) is a simple formula that combines two forms of vitamin C—ascorbic acid and tetrahexyldecyl ascorbate. Dr. Badreshia-Bansal's Powerhouse C Serum (elitemdspa.com) also combines L-ascorbic with tetrahexydecyl ascorbate, and adds green tea extract and vitamin E. Neither I nor my dermatology colleagues have any experience with Nourish Max vitamin C, B, E and ferulic serum (mourishmax.com), but it does have a 20% concentration of ascorbic acid, is well packaged and, given the active ingredient mix, is relatively inexpensive so it might be worth a try.

Other topical antioxidants to watch for:

- **Green Tea Extract.** The leaves of *Camelia sinensis* contain four polyphenols the most prevalent of which is epigallocatechin gallate (EGCG).[187] Green tea polyphenols protect against UV radiation.[188] and reduce the signs of premature skin ageing from UVB rays.[189]

- **Niacinamide.** Vitamin B3 is a powerful, well studied antioxidant that is commonly added to topical skincare products where it can help moisturize, soothe, and brighten the skin.[190,191,192] For these reasons it is often included in topical sunblocks for people who are acne-prone. You will find niacinamide in eltaMD's UV Clear Broad-Spectrum SPF 46, Color Science All Calm® SPF 50 and SkinCeuticals Clinical Redness Corrector. Niacinamide without sunblock is a key bioactive in products such as Nia 24 Intensive Recovery Complex and SkinCeuticals MetaCell Renewal B3.

  Niacinamide is also the basis for Biopelle's Emepelle®, a topical designed to improve the appearance of estrogen deficient skin. Empelle also contains other antioxidants such as vitamins C and E, camellia sinensis leaf extract, superoxide dismutase, and ferulic acid.

- **Resveratrol.** This grape-based antioxidant got a strong boost in popularity when Harvard geneticist David Sinclair, PhD, discovered that resveratrol could extend the life of mice treated with the compound.[193] Resveratrol is the antioxidant responsible for imparting the deep purple red color to wine. Lest you get too excited about the benefits this libation provides, note that red wine contains less than 2 mg of resveratrol per 150 ml. A person would have to consume about a hundred bottles of wine to approach the amount of resveratrol fed to the mice. SkinCeuticals offers a resveratrol product (Resveratrol B E) as does Caudalié, (caudalie.com) called Vinosource. Caudalié is a French product company recommended by Dr. Waldorf.

- **Algae Based Products.** If you remember back to the discussion of oral antioxidants, I noted the power of astaxanthin, the reddish pigment derived from algae. So, it makes sense that both red and blue algae are packed with antioxidants and are now being incorporated into topical skincare. There aren't many algae-based products made available by dermatologists, but you can find moderately priced products online.

PEPTIDES

Peptides are distinguished from proteins by their size and structure. Peptides are smaller than proteins, usually being made up of between 2 and 50 amino acids, while proteins are made up of 50 or more amino acids. Peptides are the building blocks of the all-important proteins, so it makes sense—if they can penetrate into the dermis where they can affect the ECM—to try to infuse them into the skin. The rate-limiting issue is size, and to some extent structure.

Growth factors are metabolically active byproducts of cells grown in culture. They are large peptide molecules, up to 100X the size of vitamin C. Growth factors differ depending upon the cell source from which they were derived. Different stem cells secrete different growth factors when cultured under different conditions. PRP, plasma rich platelets, for example, secrete a different mix of growth factors than do stem cells. Growth factors go by a set of initials such as EGF (epidermal growth factor), FGF (fibroblast growth factor), TGF-beta (transforming growth factor beta). Once inside the dermis, they exert different positive effects on the ECM.

The first use of growth factors in topical skincare was pioneered by Richard Fitzpatrick, MD, who founded SkinMedica in 1999. Fitzpatrick created the breakthrough TNS Recovery Complex® (Tissue Nutrient Solution). A few years later, the company developed a TNS Essential Serum that combined TNS Recovery Complex with antioxidants and peptides. Despite the fact that the actual mechanism of how these large growth factors get into the skin is unknown (Down the hair shaft? Through cracks in the skin?), SkinMedica products are being used by thousands of skin professionals worldwide with many patients reporting excellent results.

PEPTIDES FOR ECM MODULATION

Dr. Fitzpatrick's work kicked off an entire category of skin treatment—one that utilizes smaller peptides to penetrate the extracellular matrix in the dermis and affect both collagen and elastin.

According to Dr. Waldorf, "When I was in training, we were taught that we couldn't have an effect on the elastin. Now we know we can improve elastin as well as collagen. So younger-looking skin has different elastin than photodamaged skin." Dr. Waldorf, and several of the other dermatologists with whom I spoke, are enthusiastic about Alastin's products (alastin.com). The company's TriHex™ technology combines tripeptides and hexapeptides that together stimulate the GAGs, elastin and collagen in the ECM.[194]

The profile of these peptides and their inclusion into topicals with other ingredients make the Alastin product ideal as a pre-procedure treatment to ramp up the skin's regeneration process, as well as help the skin recover afterwards. You can think of this pre-and post-treatment as improving the "skin bed."

A number of other companies make interesting peptides. Dr. Ablon is fond of the Revox™ 7 products (revox.com). Dr. Chilukuri notes the uniqueness of DefenAge's serums (defenage.com). These products feature their age-repair defensins technology. One of the mechanisms of action of the small peptide defensins is their ability to stimulate a type of stem cell called LGR6+ that reside in the base of the hair follicles. Stimulating these stem cells increases the formation of new keratinocytes (skin cells).

Dr. Aguilera frequently recommends Revox™ Line Relaxer (revisionskincare.com) that features 5 neuromodulating peptides. According to Dr. Aguilera, "This targeted synergistic serum enhances the results of neuromodulators and at the same time improves skin health. It is best to prevent the crinkles under the eyes from lack of elasticity. This is a problem faced by people 40 and over. The delicate under eye area can look baggy and accordion-like when a person smiles. Injectable neurotoxins (like Botox®) alone can't solve all the problems when it comes to wrinkles. In fact, they can sometimes make things worse if they are used in areas of movement where there is poor quality skin."

More Good Stuff with GAGs

Another powerful ECM modulator takes advantage of a category of natural peptides bound to sugars in the skin (good sugars, that is). These modulators are called proteoglycans; *proteo* being the protein, and *glycan* referring to the sugar. Each molecule contains more protein than sugar.

While there are a number of bioactive proteoglycans, the one that has been studied the most and is the most powerful is heparan sulfate (HS). NOTE: it is not to be confused with the drug heparin. Heparan sulfate is found in all skin layers. It is an essential component of cell surfaces, helps to maintain the integrity of the basal membrane (the very bottom part of the epidermis where it joins the dermis), and aids in the renewal of stem cells. Perhaps most importantly, HS fills space in the ECM and binds water up to 1,000 times its volume.

Senté (sente.com) has created flagship products featuring HS based on the pioneering work of Richard Gallo, MD, PhD, Chairman of Dermatology at University of California San Diego.[195] In full disclosure, I was involved in performing one of the early studies in which we were able to show that the HS molecule, despite being 12X larger than vitamin C, was able to penetrate into the dermis. This is in part due to the long, thin shape of the molecule itself. I have no ongoing interest in Senté but am a big fan of their products.

Interesting, but More Research Needed

When my son—a gifted writer—was in high school, I was able to get him a job as a medical writer for THE Aesthetic Guide (theaestheticguide.com), where he interviewed leading cosmetic professionals. As he read through articles on aesthetic products, he asked me why most of the articles in the scientific literature ended with the phrase, "Promising, but further studies are needed." Most topical studies report results on small groups of patients (between 10 and 50) who are usually only followed for 4-12 weeks; hence the authors qualify their positive results by acknowledging these limitations. In that spirit, here are some of the newer ingredients trying to make their way onto the red carpet of topical products.

Probiotics

I love the skin microbiome story. It's a glimpse into the future. The search for the *right* probiotics to apply to the skin for the *right* person has captured the attention and research dollars of the major cosmeceutical manufactures. We can look forward to waves of products being introduced into the market. The reality is "It's complicated." Knowing *which* bugs, do what, in *which* environments, in *which* people; well, it's still very much trial and error. There's too much we don't know. Here are just a handful of the bacteria being studied for their specific effects on skin:

- *Bifidobacterium* to reduce skin sensitivity and boost the barrier effects of ceramides
- *Lactobacillus* to reduce acne and redness
- *Vitreoscilla* to decrease water loss from the skin
- *Bacillus coagulans* to counter free radicals
- *Streptococcus thermopolis* to aid sensitive skin

And the list could go on. The bottom line is that this is a very, very young science. I've tried LaFlore® (laflore.com), a skincare line infused with live probiotics. Their three key products contain Bifida bacteria and Lactobacillus strains, Saccharomyces, Pycnogenol® and a variety of antioxidant vitamins and minerals for gentle cleansing, moisturizing, and strengthening the skin microbiome. LaFlore® is promoted for all skin types, but they state it is especially good for sensitive, irritated, and/or rosacea-prone skin.

Mushrooms

The use of mushrooms in skincare is not new. These fungi have been used for medicinal purposes by Eastern cultures for centuries. While some researchers are exploring mushrooms' potential as oral ingredients for immune health, others are looking at how mushrooms can reduce the severity of inflammatory skin disease and correct hyperpigmentation.[196] Mushrooms contain high levels of two powerful antioxidants—glutathione and ergothioneine—that can aid in skin beauty.[197] The argument for mushrooms is further advanced by research on beta-glucan, found in mushrooms, showing improvement in the skin barrier. This can help calm irritated skin.[198]

Topical preparations now available on the market draw from multiple types of mushrooms, including chaga, turkey tail, tremella, shiitake, reishi, and cordyceps. A number of manufacturers are encapsulating their mushroom extracts to improve penetration into the skin. Those interested in mushroom-based topicals could give Dr. Andrew Weil for Origins™ (origins.com) or Dr. Dennis Gross's products a try (drdennisgross.com).

Cannabis

I consider cannabis a product in search of a market. Over the last few years, we've witnessed the explosion of legalized marijuana and hemp-based products. There's been a mad scramble to find products into which manufacturers can insert cannabinoids (active molecules in hemp). I'm a fan of understanding the endocannabinoid system—which describes a set of receptors throughout the body—but without a solid mechanism of action and data on efficacy, I'd advise you not to count on cannabis-based ingredients being anywhere near the effectiveness for skin beauty as the other ingredients mentioned previously.

Physician-Branded Topicals

Earlier I mentioned the important role physicians play in formulating and testing skincare products. Some practitioners get so passionate about the need for clean (sensitizing-free), efficacious formulations, that they go about launching their own proprietary brands. They make these products available for sale on their websites.

Dr. Doris Day (dorisdaymd.com) first got excited about topicals early in her career, when as a researcher at NYU, she studied the effects of vitamin A and other antioxidants on skin cells. As one of the most prominent dermatologists in the NYC area, it was only natural that leading skincare companies would seek her input on their product formulation. While the large companies create excellent products, Dr. Day identified many patients who were not well served through the mass market.

One example is the need to address skin issues caused by constant mask wearing, an aesthetic issue Dr. Day addressed by creating her All Day Masque Serum. Describing her rationale she notes, "The microbes from the mouth often end up causing a breakout in the area around the mouth. The skin becomes compromised from wearing a mask for extended periods of time. The type of skin breakdown and breakout that follows is a very specific rash–different from acne or rosacea and it needs to be treated in a specific and unique way." Her topicals have the benefit of being well sourced, high value ingredients, each of which has a synergistic and additive effect on the other.

NOTE: On minimizing mask-related acne, I'd also recommend a probiotic designed to optimize the composition of the oral bacteria. Immune Max™ Immuno-Biotic Defense Mints (enzymedica.com) were created by Japanese researchers who have a long history of dealing with mask wearing. The mints deliver 12 billion cells of clinically studied HKL-137 Probiotic. The quick melt in the mouth provides the same, nice burst of mint as breath fresheners, but with a healthy dose of probiotics. An interesting finding, in an animal study, Japanese researchers have also shown this same probiotic upregulates collagen production for extra skin support.[199]

Epionce® (epionce.com) is the brainchild of Carl Thornfeldt, MD, a dermatologist who teamed up with a noted chemist in 2002 to create this product line. Highly regarded for his talks on topicals, I place enormous faith in his views on skin science. I personally love the smell and feel of these products. Three other clinician-developed product lines worthy of investigation are the recently-launched Soyier™ Skin Collection (gfacemd.com) created by Harvard-trained dermatopathologist Gretchen Frieling, MD. I haven't tried the products, but I enjoy watching her teach on social media. Healthcare professionals Jill Carnahan, MD (drjillhealth.com) and Sahar Swidan, PharmD (sahar.world) lean on their functional medicine training in creating skin care formulas that incorporate nice blends of antioxidants and other nutrients and leave out harmful additives.

Personalized Skincare: It Depends
I confess I got a bit of payback for my frequent "It depends" comment when I asked each of the dermatologists, "What should a person apply to their skin?"

The docs' universal response, "It depends." As professionals, they distinguish between wrinkles caused by excessive facial muscle movement (requiring neuromodulators), fine lines and wrinkles. They assess pigment, redness, veins, and potential skin cancers. They get a sense for laxity, deflation, and loss of elasticity in the face. All of this takes place so that they can make specific recommendations for each individual based upon:

- **Skin conditions.** Recommendations for an older patient with extensive photodamage will be significantly different from those provided to a 30-something looking to begin an anti-aging skin regimen.

- **Complexity versus simplicity of routine.** Unless there is irritation, most people don't need a separate product for every body part. Not everyone needs a serum, although these tend to be well accepted by men who don't like the greasier feel of some products.

- **Natural versus science-based preferences.** It's your choice, based upon your beliefs. If you feel more aligned with nature, look for products based on infused oils, and all herbal extracts. Like and believe in science? You've got so many great choices.

- **Affordability.** There are many great products on the market produced by some of the larger and smaller companies. Olay® Regenerist has plenty of science to back it up, as do Avène and Neutrogena®. All of these are moderately priced. If you believe that there is incremental value in more expensively priced products, and you see consistent results, go with, and stick with these products.

- **Prioritization.** Ultimately, you'll need to determine what's most important to do in order to have beautiful skin. Yes, the right topicals help, but there's little that you can do to rescue the skin devastation caused by a crappy diet and unrelenting environmental exposure.

> ## THE VEXING PROBLEM OF PIGMENT
>
> Smaller pigmented sun-induced spots respond well to IPL and laser treatments. They can be noticeably lightened by topicals that contain high-concentrations of antioxidants or other compounds such as kojic acid, a byproduct of malted rice. The exception is melasma that's deeply seated in the dermis. Melasma is a chronic hormonally-induced pigmentation problem most common in women who have had children. It usually recedes in winter and flares up in the hot months. The diffuse brown pigment usually presents symmetrically as classic butterflies under the cheeks, or patches on the forehead or chin. Melasma tends to be more pronounced in people of Hispanic and Asian heritage. Although frequent, very low-level laser treatments are often used to help curtail it, there really is no cure. In addition to the antioxidant topicals noted, manufacturers are producing skin brightening agents that can help with generalized pigment. One of these is Cyspera® by Senté. It contains cysteamine, a powerful antioxidant. Another skin brightening product is SkinMedica's Lytera® Pigment Correcting Serum that contains niacinamide, tetrapeptide-30, and tranexamic acid.

Do As I Do, and Do What I Say

Go ahead and do an image search on the dermatologists I've profiled. You'll see they all have gorgeous skin. No surprises there. Sure, it's easy to attribute their pulchritude to the fact that they have easy and "free" access to aesthetic devices, injectables, and age-defying topicals. But I assure you: with the exception of one of the docs, I've spent time with each and enjoyed more than one meal with them. If you were to watch how and what they eat, and the attention they pay to their diet, you'd get a real sense of how they walk the talk when it comes to the nutritional choices they make.

One example: In the course of interviewing Dr. Ablon over Zoom, I saw a mason jar containing a brown liquid near her desk. When I asked what it was, she told me it was her breakfast beauty juice, whose recipe is included on the next page.

Dr. Ablon's Breakfast Beauty Drink
(All ingredients are organic)
- 1/2 grapefruit
- 1/2 avocado
- 1 tbsp chia seeds (soaked overnight)
- 3x3cm bar of cacao butter
- 1 tsp cacao nibs
- 1 raw egg
- 1 handful of lingonberries, elderberries, sea buckthorn (frozen but organic) about 1/3 of each
- 1 tsp juiced turmeric root
- 1 tsp raw ginger juiced to make puree
- Mountain Valley Spring Water (to fill mason jar)

When patients comment on her concoction, and make remarks like, "Oh, I don't like avocados," or "I don't like grapefruits," her response is simple. "So? I don't like everything I eat, but I do like what it does for my health and skin." I rest my case on the synergistic power of diet and bioactive topicals. Let's now turn to how selected injectables and aesthetic devices create healthy skin from the inside out.

Part Four: What Procedures Should I Have?

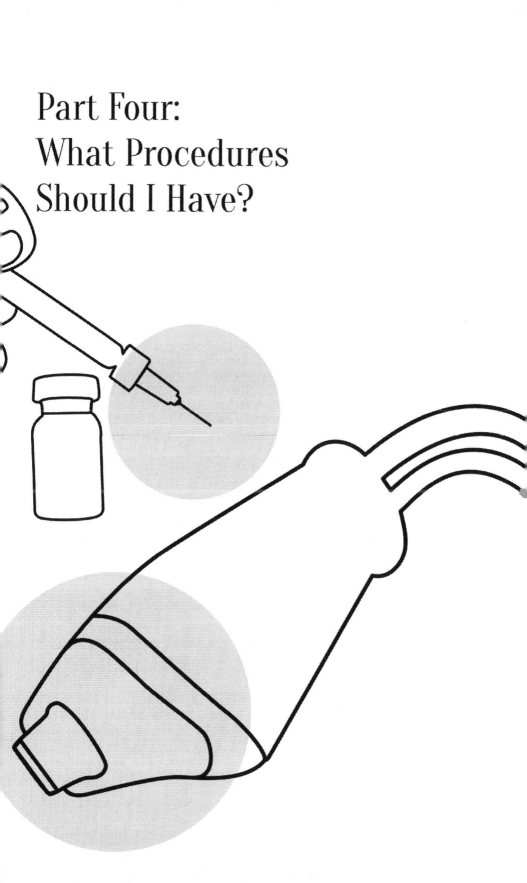

"The laser is only as good as the provider using it."

Lori Robertson, NP

Chapter 13

AESTHETIC DEVICES, INJECTABLES & YOUR SKIN

What's Ahead

Keeping in the spirit of this book, I'll confine our discussion of devices and injectables to products and procedures that stimulate the dermis to create healthy skin from within (biostimulation). This is not to discount the superficial beauty-enhancing procedures that affect just the epidermis, such as light peels, microdermabrasion, or hydrodermabrasion; or the spot removal of brown pigments or unsightly blood vessels. These procedures all have a place in creating superficial beauty. I also will not be discussing neurotoxins such as Botox®, Dysport®, or Xeomin®. Neuromodulators are valuable agents for looking younger, but their effects are purely mechanical—softening the appearance of muscle-driven wrinkles.

AESTHETIC DEVICES 101

To choose the type of device treatment that will work best to stimulate your skin, there are a few key concepts you'll want to understand.

Collagen Remodeling. Collagen is a tightly coiled molecule in the dermis. When it is subjected to the right amount of heat for a certain time, it unwinds and shortens. It essentially becomes inert and signals the ECM to create new collagen (neocollagenesis). The old, inactivated collagen becomes the scaffold upon which the new collagen is created, a shaping process known as remodeling. Depending upon the procedure, this remodeling can go on for as long as six months. The full beneficial effects of a procedure may not be observed until this time. The ability to remodel collagen decreases with age. While nutrition plays a big role for any one individual, in general, people in their 30s, 40s, and mid-50s will obtain greater/faster collagen-enhancing benefits than those in their more advanced years.

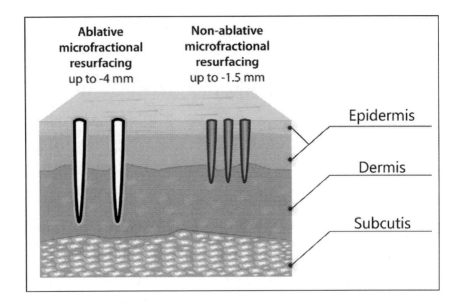

Fractional Treatment. My colleagues pioneered this approach to skin resurfacing when we developed the Fraxel® laser in the early 2000s. It involves the creation of small channels in the skin, with healthy skin left in between. It is called "fractional" because only a percentage of the skin is actually wounded. The unaffected skin participates in rapid healing. The channels are less than the width of a hair follicle, almost invisible to the naked eye. In any given treatment, usually only 10-20% of the skin is directly involved. However, when laser or radiofrequency (RF) heat is applied, the heat can spread in the dermis and help accelerate the collagen remodeling process throughout the treated skin. Most recently, microneedling is being used to create these fractional channels. When it is combined with RF energy, the microneedling can deliver heat into the dermis. Many aesthetic device companies now offer machines that perform RF Microneedling.

Ablative versus Non-Ablative. These terms usually apply to two different types of laser actions that depend upon the wavelength being used. In an ablative procedure, the tissue is vaporized. This can occur either fractionally, or the laser can be used to carefully remove the entire top layer of the skin. A non-ablative laser uses a wavelength that coagulates the tissue. It turns it into a more gel-like substance that then stimulates the body to heal the wound by creating newer skin. In either case, the old dead skin will slough off several days after the procedure. For maximum results, most non-ablative treatments, and all microneedling treatments, will require multiple sessions spaced out over time. Ablative fractional resurfacing (usually with a CO_2 laser) is a one-time treatment that temporarily (24 hours or less) creates open channels into the skin. The trade-off between ablative versus non-ablative laser treatment is downtime.

Device-Topical Combinations. The energy-based procedures that breach the skin barrier present an opportunity to deliver biostimulants (regenerative molecules) into the skin. The skin doesn't normally allow for much penetration of these larger molecules. With the skin more open to penetration, some aesthetic practitioners are applying biostimulants at the time of treatment, or are instructing patients to self-apply topicals with growth factors, antioxidants, or brightening agents.

Some physicians will recommend the application of "autologous" regenerative factors. These are cells or tissue taken from your body (auto), separated into active ingredients, and returned back to you. During the procedure your clinician will coat your face with the biostimulants in hopes of getting them to penetrate deeper into the skin. The two most commonly applied autologous topicals are PRP (isolated platelet rich plasma obtained via venipuncture at the time of procedure), and nanosized fat molecules (harvested by a syringe usually from abdominal fat). In both cases, the physician separates out the active components before applying them to your skin. The Vampire Facial™ is an example of applying PRP over the channels created by microneedling.

Procedures can also be paired with topical application of growth factor serums or exosomes, small encapsulated signaling proteins derived from stem cells.[200]

A Word about Exosomes

At this point, there are no major studies showing that application of bioactive topicals at the point of care or shortly thereafter have any major effect beyond that of the device alone. If your practitioner makes this recommendation, you would be relying on their knowledge and clinical experience to guide you.

THE FDA & EXOSOMES

The FDA has some issues with intravenous and injectable exosomes, noting they are: "concerned that many patients seeking cures and remedies may be misled by information about products that are illegally marketed, have not been shown to be safe or effective, and, in some cases, may have significant safety issues that put patients at risk." At present, their concern does not seem to cross over into general topical use for exosome products; however, the FDA may be more wary about the possibility of introducing these proteins directly into the dermis in conjunction with minimally invasive procedures.[201]

Energy Sources. The principle behind most aesthetic device treatments is to "wound" the body, thereby stimulating the healing response and creating younger skin. For energy devices, the different sources include Intense Pulsed Light (Think of a giant flash lamp with different filters to address pigment or redness.), lasers, radiofrequency, ultrasound, plasma (an electrostatic mixture of oxygen and nitrogen arced over the skin), or cold (cryotherapy). Energies that penetrate deeper into the dermis are more likely to result in skin tightening in patients who have good capacity to remodel their collagen. RF and focused ultrasound are two of the major modalities for skin tightening. Lasers powered by CO_2 can deeply penetrate the skin where the CO_2 rays vaporize water and create enough heat in the dermis to activate proteins that can result in skin tightening. Deeper microneedling procedures manually disrupt the skin, which repairs itself through increased collagen and elastin formation. Home-based microneedling devices are limited to only penetrating the epidermis; professional devices can reach the dermis.

With Low-level Light Therapy (LLLT), the skin absorbs certain wavelengths (usually red and blue light). This stimulates the energy-producing mitochondria in the skin cells, as well as increases nitric oxide release and blood flow. The original light sources were lasers. Now LLLT is usually done via the much safer light emitting diodes (LEDs). With safety established, companies are now making these devices available direct to consumers. LightStim (lightstim.com) produces a quality line of LLTs to counter skin aging and other issues. Like nutraceuticals and topicals, the results are subtle, require regular use, and take time to become observable.[202]

Another interesting technology that has an anti-aging component is EMSculpt (EMSculpt.com) This device uses electromagnetic energy to contract and strengthen muscles beyond what is possible with voluntary effort. While it is used exclusively on the body, the metabolism-enhancing effects of this stimulation have benefits beyond just muscle strengthening. To account for the increase in energy required by the muscles, nearby fat cells break up, donating their energy to feed the muscular activity. The result is increased muscle tone and less fat, a winning prescription for most Americans. When radiofrequency is added to the device, the fat loss is accelerated.

Safety. The good news is that most of the lasers have gotten much safer over the years. In the hands of well-trained, experienced users who provide thorough informed consent, you should be comfortable that you are in good hands. One of the touchiest areas involves using energy devices on individuals with darker skin types. This can result in post inflammatory hyperpigmentation (PIH) which primarily affects darker skin types, particularly people with Hispanic or Asian heritage. The skin becomes inflamed because it absorbs too much heat from this treatment, and the increased inflammation stimulates melanin production. The result is excess brown pigment after the treatment.

NOTE: People with melasma need to be extra cautious about avoiding any laser or energy device (IPL, ablative and non-ablative lasers) that delivers heat to the skin. This can trigger a flare up of the pigment. Aesthetic professionals go through a standard process in assessing skin health and beauty. They begin by assigning the patient a skin type based upon how much sun the skin can tolerate. This scale—known as the Fitzpatrick scale—correlates with the amount of pigment in the skin, hence it is more widely thought of as a measure of skin color. The Fitzpatrick scale also alerts the clinician to the energy settings that can be safely used with aesthetic devices for the different skin types. Invasive type procedures are contraindicated in people who tend to develop keloids, raised fibrous scars caused by abnormal collagen remodeling.

> ## FITZPATRICK SKIN TYPES
> **Type I** – always burns, never tans (palest; tends to get freckles)
> **Type II** – usually burns, tans minimally (light colored but darker than fair)
> **Type III** – sometimes mild burn, tans uniformly (golden honey or olive)
> **Type IV** – burns minimally, always tans well (moderate brown)
> **Type V** – very rarely burns, tans very easily (dark brown)
> **Type VI** – never burns (deeply pigmented dark brown to darkest brown)

Downtime. The amount of downtime needed is a result of the type and strength of energy used, the depth of penetration, and in the case of fractional treatment, how closely the channels are placed together. However, there are always outliers—people who for some reason, take much longer to recover from a procedure. We don't know why this occurs.

Generally, most fractional ablative laser procedures take 5-9 days to totally heal. This occurs when all the old, treated skin flakes off. Most people are able to resume their daily activities days earlier, looking as if they just had a sunburn. The remaining redness depends on the depth and strength of the treatment. The general axiom is that "the longer the downtime, the better the outcome." In contrast to lasers, IPL and microneedling (without RF) have shorter healing times.

To best set patient expectations, E. Victor Ross, MD, a San Diego based dermatologist who specializes in laser surgery of the skin, shows photographs of patients who have undergone the recommended procedure at different time points (i.e. immediately after, day 1, day 3, day 7). Ask your clinician if they have similar photographs.

Cost. There are many factors that go into the cost of a procedure, beyond the practitioner's time and overhead. Most clinics lease their devices and pay for them over time. Price points must also account for any disposable costs to use the device. For some devices, practitioners must buy tips, or pay to use time on their devices. These costs can represent anywhere from

5-20% of what you ultimately pay. Increasingly, clinics are offering patient financing for the more expensive procedures.

Pain. Discomfort accompanies all aesthetic procedures, whether they are devices or injectables. Fortunately, through the use of cold packs, devices that blow cold air over the skin, topical application of numbing medications, and the inhalation of nitrous oxide laughing gas (Pro-Nox™), you should be comfortable during treatment. If your clinician instructs you to arrive for your appointment early (usually 40 minutes to 1 hour) for numbing, don't cut this time short. You want to have a very tolerable experience. Generally, after many procedures, your skin will feel like you've got a sunburn which will subside in several hours. Make certain to let your practitioner know if you have any allergies to the numbing medicines (lidocaine, benzocaine, tetracaine, etc.).

What to Look for in Your Clinician

How do you find a good injector? A clinician with a measured eye for beauty? Someone who listens to you and addresses your primary concerns? An injector who is experienced, well-trained, and places safety above everything else? You can ask friends for referrals, peruse websites, examine credentials, look at reviews, view practitioner videos, and check online for any available before and after photographs. These are all helpful steps, but nothing takes the place of a thoughtful consultation. In the consultation, you are looking and listening for your provider's understanding of three things:

- **The anatomy of the face.** The best injectors have a thorough understanding of facial anatomy. Many take specialized cadaver classes to enhance their skill. Every injectable procedure carries a measure of risk. At the least, it will be predictable bruising or swelling; at the worst, it can be a serious complication related to injecting the wrong substance in the wrong place. Plastic surgeons have the most thorough understanding of anatomy; however, they are not necessarily the best injectors. Dermatologists, and licensed extenders (NPs, PAs, RNs) usually have the most experience.

    When you have discussions with your practitioner, ask them to explain the procedure from an anatomical perspective. Ask why they have chosen the specific product for each area of your face and where it will be placed. Listen carefully for their answers. You should come away with a good understanding of the rationale behind and location of the filler placement.

- **The physiology of aging.** Unfortunately, aging is a symphony in which bony structures, fat pads, and each skin layer participates in a rather depressing adagio. While there's no way to stop the deterioration, you can slow it down. That's the role of the biostimulant fillers. They stimulate your body to make collagen and elastin or fat to replace the natural tissue loss. The best practitioners work with you to create an anatomically sound plan based upon how you are aging. They recognize what's within their scope of ability—with the materials they have in hand—and when to refer you for surgery.

- **The mechanism of action of the injectables** (what they do, how long they last). A professional is going to inject a substance into your face which may or may not contain the same ingredients as your own tissue. It is their responsibility—as well as yours—to thoroughly understand how the filler will contribute to skin health and beauty. We'll now turn our attention to exploring this.

HOW FILLERS WORK

Lori Robertson, NP, who practices in Brea, California, is one of the most skilled injectors in the country. In addition to training for two major injectable manufacturers Galderma and Allergan, she also runs a teaching academy for professionals (theasetheticimmersion.com). In discussions with her patients, she makes the distinction between two classifications of fillers:
- Fillers that revolumize with tissue expansion, and
- Biostimulants that regenerate tissue.

Revolumization. I liken these fillers to blowing up a balloon. The most commonly used revolumization agent is hyaluronic acid (HA). Hyaluronic acid is one of the natural sponges that attracts and holds water. The five different brands available in the US (Juvéderm®, Restylane® Belotero®, Revanesse®, and RHA®) offer a spectrum of HA fillers manufactured to either provide more structure or more fluidity. Europe has many more approved HA fillers. The clinician decides which product is the best to use in a specific area of the face. While the filler is present, there is volume.

The common wisdom is that the HA fillers last for six months to a year; however, Robertson notes work done by Dr. Gavin Chan, MBBS, founder of Victorian Cosmetic Institute, showing that small amounts of injected HA can be detected in MRIs in some patients for additional years. HA longevity is often very variable. Robertson believes this may be due to the different rates at which people's natural hyaluronidase breaks down the filler.

Regardless, when the majority of the HA is gone, the balloon (your skin) becomes deflated. There is no stimulation of the dermis. The skin itself is not being stretched out of shape, so when the filler is no longer present, the skin will go back to where it was before you started (plus the changes of normal aging). From a purely cometic standpoint, one of the major advantages of HA fillers is the ability to dissolve any unsightly lumps or overfilled areas with an injectable enzyme called hyaluronidase.[203]

Biostimulants. These products stimulate the body's natural production of collagen, and to a lesser extent, may affect elastin. They fall into two categories, the first of which includes the non-HA fillers, the second involves the regenerative fillers. Regenerative fillers (often called biofilling) take advantage of using biological material either from you or from a donor and injecting it into your skin.

BIOSTIMULANT PRODUCTS (NON-HA)
- **Radiesse®** – The injection of calcium hydroxylapatite (CaHA) microspheres initially provides volume. Over time, the gel filler stimulates the body's own production of collagen. When injected above the bone and under the dermis (subdermis), Radiesse has shown improvement in tightening and elastin formation over 18 months or more.[204] Unlike hyaluronic acids, this product is not dissolvable should there be a problem with placement.

    One of the newer applications of Radiesse involves diluting it so that it forms a thin whipped cream-like substance which can then be easily injected. When diluted, Radiesse no longer has a volumizing effect, but acts as a biostimulant for more superficial dermal rejuvenation and treatment of larger areas.[205,206]

- **Bellafill®** is a semi-permanent filler with results that can last up to five years. It achieves this through stimulating collagen with tiny polymethyl methacrylate (PMMA) microspheres that are suspended in a smooth collagen gel. One of the challenges of such a long-lasting filler has to do with placement. Robertson cautions that, "As the face ages and takes on different shapes, the filler remains in the same place. and this can contribute to an unnatural appearance."[207] Similar to Radiesse, semi-permanent fillers are not reversible.

- **Sculptra®** – Hands down this is one of the favorite biostimulants of my dermatologic colleagues. Sculptra Aesthetic is injectable poly-L-lactic acid. When placed down near the bone it provides ongoing stimulation for deep collagen build-up. When injected in the cheeks or temple areas it provides both volume and ongoing stimulation. According to Lori Robertson, "Sculptra is best used for 'pan-facial' volume loss. We use it in places where other fillers would look too unnatural or firm, especially because we would need to inject large amounts of these other fillers." The most noticeable results can be observed for up to two years. Once formed, the Sculptra-stimulated collagen degrades along with the body's natural collagen over time. Most often a series of injections are required, usually 4-6 weeks apart. Younger patients generally see results more quickly than older patients.

REGENERATIVE PRODUCTS

Platelet Rich Plasma (PRP).[208,209,210] Earlier I discussed the use of PRP in hair restoration and as a topical applied to microneedling. Platelet rich plasma is prepared by removing a small quantity of your blood and then spinning it down to separate out the platelet growth factors. The growth factor mix can then be injected into the skin where it works as a modest biostimulant that mainly helps improve skin texture. The difficulty with assessing the clinical results from PRP is two-fold. Not only is there variability in the quality of PRP with aging, but there's also no consistent collection system. The larger studies on PRP compile all the different approaches. Without standardization, it's difficult to make any intelligent comparisons as to what works. PRP may also be combined with Autologous Fat Transfer.

Autologous Fat. This is your fat ("Auto") that is being extracted, purified, and injected back into you. Usually, a small amount of fat is harvested from the flanks, or abdomen, micronized (made into smaller fractions), and then reinjected into your face, neck, hands or décolletage. The procedure can be done in office under local anesthesia or done in a surgical suite with sedation. The purified fat is a rich mix of stem cells, exosomes and growth factors with potent biostimulatory properties.

Steven Cohen, MD, a plastic surgeon and clinical professor at UCSD, is my go-to doc for all questions related to fat grafting. Autologous fat transfer has been around for more than twenty years. The earliest results were very variable; without properly preparing the fat so that it will "take", most patients only retained 20-40%. Dr. Cohen is one of the pioneers of techniques to improve the extraction and preparation of fat. He considers fat to be a natural filler, not an alternative. Citing a soon-to-be published study of 30 patients, he notes that the best results are seen in patients under 55 years old. "In these younger patients, we have maintained an 80% improvement of facial volume after 2 years. This drops down to a 30% improvement in patients over 55 years of age."

Renuva® is a fat replacement that is available as an injectable. It is fairly new on the market, and somewhat costly, but it eliminates the need for harvesting your own fat. Renuva acquires its material from cadavers. Now, before you go, "Ugh" at the thought of injecting cadaver tissue into your body, consider that allogeneic (from someone else) tissue has been used for decades to replace tendons and ligaments, or to replace bone in surgical or dental procedures. The tissue banks from which fat is derived, sterilize the fat and purify it to remove any DNA. What is left is the fat scaffold, which when injected in an area where you want fat (like replaces like), does two things. It immediately replaces volume, but more importantly, it also stimulates the stem cells to fill in the fat scaffold with your own fat. This process is similar to how collagen gets remodeled. The best results from the procedure occur several months out. Because Renuva is regulated as an HCT/P[211] (human cells, tissues, and cellular tissue-based product) it has not gone through the same large-scale safety and efficacy trials that the FDA mandates for other fillers.

Fillers on the Horizon

Collagen has received outsized attention, overshadowing perhaps its more important bedfellow—elastin. Elastin fibers provide the stretch, recoil, and elasticity to the skin. With aging, these fibers diminish. There are nutrients that can slow the rate of this deterioration, most notably. Zinc, Co-Q10, and derivatives of vitamin A. But for people with wounds, stretch marks, and scars, and for anti-aging in general, a treatment that can create elastin (elastogenesis) would be a major breakthrough.

Elastogenesis is a complex process that involves the crosslinking of a molecule called tropoelastin. Promising research is showing that injecting tropoelasin into the dermis can increase the number and thickness of elastin fibers, and generate elastin fibers regardless of age.[212] Keep your eyes open for injectables that directly promote elastogenesis.

Expectations, Impatience and Urgency

No matter what type of procedure you undergo, you'll need to make certain that your expectations are realistic. You'll also want to temper the sense of impatience and urgency that underlies your motivation to seek treatment. It takes time to see the full effects of many of the biostimulatory/regenerative treatments. There's a reason that the best aesthetic practitioners take high-quality photographs before and after treatments. You likely look at your face in the mirror multiple times a day and because the changes are taking place gradually, you may not notice the improvement. Other people who haven't seen you in a while will.

Part Five:
Your Personal Plan

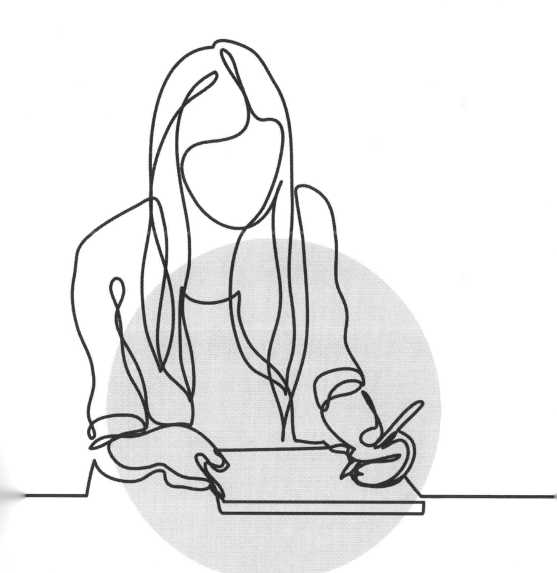

"I think your whole life shows in your face and you should be proud of that."

Lauren Bacall

Chapter 14

WHAT'S *RIGHT* FOR YOU

I hope you've enjoyed your journey through *Feed Your Skin Right*. In the introduction I covered the importance of "turning on the light" and making the connection between what you eat and how you feel. I also shared my own story of personal wellness transformation, and detailed why I changed my diet and lifestyle habits. Each of us is on an individual path to health and beauty. Just as there are unique needs for nutrients, topicals, and procedures, so too are there individual steps to making healthy changes. The goal is to find what's right for you in terms of creating *your* personalized plan. There are six factors you must take into account; these are the variables upon which your health and beauty depend.

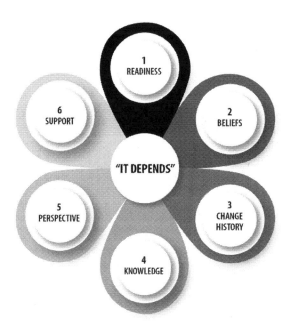

Readiness. One of the major theories of health behavior change was advanced by psychologist James Prochaska, PhD, who coined the Stages of Change or Transtheoretical Model. It consists of five stages, beginning with Precontemplation (in which you are not aware of the need for change). Since you picked up this book, you've advanced to at least the Contemplation stage, which is then followed by Preparation (getting ready for change), Action, and finally Maintenance.

I've always found a few things helpful for people to move through these stages. The first is to get absolutely clear on your motivations and willingness to change your lifestyle and diet. You want to have radiant skin, sure, but what else? Ease aches and pains? Live longer? Be gorgeous/handsome for a big event? Gain energy? Attract a new significant other?

Another thing is to start small. Pick the one thing that you will absolutely do, no matter what. Make it easy, bite-sized, and attainable. For example, try time restricted feeding for a week; see how you feel, and determine how easy it might be to incorporate into your routine longer term. Cut out simple carbohydrates for a week? Consume more olive oil, avocados, or flax? Grow some veggies indoors or outside? Slip resistance exercises into your daily routine? You get the idea. Flip back through the pages of *FYSR* and find the one thing you are going to *start* doing; one thing you are going to *stop* doing; and one thing you're doing well that you'll *keep* doing. The secret is to get an early "win," and then move on from there to setting more challenging goals.

Beliefs. When it comes to nutrition, and creating a personalized plan, it's a bit like religion. People have deeply instilled, powerfully held beliefs about what to eat, and what not to eat. On one hand we have the paleo diet, heavy in meat protein; on the other we have vegetarianism and vegan diets. A plant-centered diet is great for health and beauty, but if you are going to rely very heavily on it to the exclusion of dairy, meat, and fish, you'll need to be ever vigilant to get all the nutrients you need from food. Vegans will need to supplement with B12, vitamin D, omega 3-fatty acids, iron for menstruating women and most likely zinc.

The most important belief is known as empowerment, often referred to by psychologists as the "locus of control." To empower yourself, you must believe you have the power to make positive changes. Many years ago, when I was Director of Health Promotion for the Northwest Region at Kaiser Permanente, we did an all-employee survey, asking respondents, "If you really wanted to make a major change in your behavior, could you do it?" Interestingly, the overwhelming majority, greater than 90% said they could. The follow-up question was, "If you were to make this major change, would it make a difference in your health?" Only about 3% said, it wouldn't make any difference; perhaps they were too far gone, or too cynical. But for the vast majority the belief was there, albeit at different levels. You'll just want to strengthen and reinforce your power of control with visualizations, daily meditations, prayer, affirmations and the encouragement of positive people in your life.

Change History. When I used to counsel patients on changing their yo-yo dieting behaviors, I would often open my discussion by stating the following: "You already know exactly how you are going to sabotage your plan. Let's discuss this and come up with a way to deal with it."

Here's where you'll want to acknowledge that there will be times when you slip back. The goal of a long-term health and beauty plan is to catch yourself sooner when you slip back. For example, I have a personal rule to never let more than three days elapse without a solid exercise session including aerobics and weight training.

Knowledge. To continue with a plan, it really helps to have data. As we've shown, the best data come from multiple sources: a detailed physical exam, appropriate lab work including any necessary specialty tests, and data relating to your nutrigenomics, microbiome, and food sensitivities.

When you have a baseline of objective measurements, you can observe how the changes you are making result in better biomarkers, and this can keep you on the path to better health. Some of the most popular wellness tracking apps for consumers include MyFitnessPal, Apple Health, Apple Fitness+, Fitbit Coach, FiiT, Fooducate, Sleep Cycle, Headspace, Nudge, Lifesum, and Skincare Routine.

Perspective. All of us have what I call the commitment gap. It is the distance between what you value (**I Value**) and what you do (**I Do**).

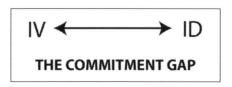

Whenever I ask people to raise their hand if they agree with the following statement, "I value my health," all the hands in the room go up. Then I ask for a show of hands by asking, "How many of you lead a life that is in perfect unison with that belief? Everything you do reflects this deeply held belief." Every hand goes down.

The best healthcare clinicians are taught to use a technique called motivational interviewing. As the name implies, this skills-based program focuses on identifying a patient's deeply seated reasons for change. Practitioners are taught listening skills and how to rework their interviewing to include more open-ended questions. The overarching goal of this process is to surface "ambivalence." In my model, ambivalence is the commitment gap between your values and actions. Every time you get your values and your actions in sync, you'll feel better and become more powerful, and others will see this coherence reflected in your body posture, gestures, tone of voice, energy, and radiance.

Support. Hopefully you are not spending too much time with people who sabotage your healthy eating habits. I've seen this way too often in couples, when one of the partners chooses to make significant, meaningful health and nutrition changes, while the other does not. This reticence can lead to subtle undermining. You'll want to choose your friends well, but equally importantly, there are times when each of us can benefit from professional guidance. Having met with, listened to, studied from, and referred patients to a small army of integrative nutrition and aesthetic professionals, I have some thoughts and recommendations on this process.

The Role of Professional Guidance

There is a large, growing movement of do-it-yourself health, facilitated by biometric technology, ease of online access, the growth of telehealth, and the ability for consumers to order tests online. For many people, signing up with a service such as Let's Get Checked or Everlywell may be all they need to make progress on their health and beauty program.

For most everyone else (and a good percentage of the DIY folks), I believe you will be best served by forging relationships with professionals who can guide you throughout your lifespan. You want someone to be invested in your health; and I'm not sure if the transactional model from many of the commercial companies will stand the test of time. The question then becomes. Whom should I look for? And, as a subsequent question, can I get everything I need from just one practitioner, or must I see multiple professionals?

For the most part, today it's a rarity to find one practitioner who can meet both your internal health needs and your external beauty wants. When it comes to whole person healthcare, you can find clinicians who go by the designation of functional, anti-aging, integrative, or holistic practitioners. Regardless of the nomenclature, these whole-person-oriented physicians will discuss the root-cause concept of disease. They'll gather the necessary data including a nutrition-oriented history and physical, basic bloodwork, and they will conduct nutrigenomics, microbiome, and food sensitivity testing. They will create a treatment plan that recognizes the primacy of lifestyle and nutrition to promote health and prevent disease. The same practitioner may or may not have cosmetic treatment skills; or they may have someone in their practice who does. Regardless, I do believe that every healthcare professional should reinforce the importance of sun protection, hydration, basic skin care, and topical treatments for common skin conditions.

Whole Person Healthcare Professional Wanted: Where to Start

For whole person healthcare, you will be best served by finding a physician who has received training from one of three organizations:

- Institute for Functional Medicine (IFM.org)
- American Academy of Anti-Aging Medicine (A4M.com)
- Academy of Integrative Health & Medicine (AIHM.org)

Each of these organizations conducts rigorous training programs featuring the philosophical approach and types of assessments and treatments I've highlighted in *FYSR*. You can search the "Find a Provider" feature of their websites to find a clinician near you. You can also schedule telehealth visits with most of these professionals if you decide you'd like to work with someone out of your area.

Another excellent option is to seek the guidance of a Naturopathic Doctor (ND). Licensed in 22 states, the DC, Puerto Rico, and US Virgin Islands, they are graduates from 4-year programs at institutions such as Bastyr University, The Southwest College of Naturopathic Medicine & Health Sciences, and the National University of Natural Medicine. NDs are trained in functional approaches to wellness and receive extensive training in personalized nutrition. You can search the American Association of Naturopathic Physicians (naturopath.org) to find a licensed naturopath near you.

Wanted: A Personalized Nutrition Professional

Here's the problem: depending on the state in which you live, anyone can call themselves a nutritionist. This means that a personal trainer, or even an interested and knowledgeable consumer, can do so; they just can't say they are state licensed or certified. They may or may not hold a certificate from a for-profit company. When it comes to wellness and nutrition, there is no shortage of initials after many people's names. There are three specialty boards that certify nutritionists and provide the credentials that help assure a level of knowledge and competence. Look for these credentials:

- **Certified Nutrition Specialist (CNS®)**. A person who holds a CNS degree is a qualified nutritional professional with an advanced degree in nutrition (graduate or doctorate) from a fully accredited university. They have completed 1,000 plus hours of a supervised internship and must pass a rigorous exam. The CNS designation is the most widely recognized nutrition certification by federal and state governments.

- **Certified Clinical Nutritionist (CCN)**. A CCN is a highly qualified nutritional professional who holds a 4-year bachelor's degree and has completed a 900-hour internship. CCNs go through significant graduate education often including a master's degree.

- **Registered Dietitian (RD)**. An RD is a food and dietary professional, usually with a 4-year bachelor's degree and 900-1200 hours in a dietetic internship. Many dieticians work in health institutions as clinical dieticians. If you choose to work with an RD, make certain that they are up to speed on the latest science in personalized healthcare as it relates to nutrition.

The list of professionals above is not to discount that there are many other licensed health and wellness professionals who have studied the discipline of personalized nutrition. They may come from the ranks of nursing, chiropractic, diabetes education, psychology, or physical therapy. It's just harder for you (and me too) to gauge the extent to which they have broadened their education beyond their formal training. Ask where they have acquired their specialized knowledge, what it entailed, and how long it took.

NOTE for Professionals: In early 2022, the American Nutrition Association (theana.org) launched its Personalized Nutrition for Practitioner certification program. Under the auspices of the Board for the Certification of Nutrition Specialists (one of the three national certification organizations), the course features 40-hours of online continuing education training. To be designated a Certified Personalized Nutrition Practitioner (CPN-P) participants must submit a case study and pass the certification exam.

Getting More from Your Aesthetic Professional

The next time you go see your aesthetic professional, ask them a simple question: "What do you think about diet and supplements?" If you have a great medical aesthetician, cosmetic practitioner, dermatologist, or plastic surgeon, they have already anticipated this question and asked about your diet, food preparation habits, and supplement use. They may have asked you to bring the supplements you currently take to your visit. These practitioners have learned the basics of a skin-inside beauty approach. They also have a well-used referral list to send their patients for functional medicine and specialty nutrition guidance.

Some clinicians will carry professional-grade supplements in their office, assuring you of quality and safety. Others will encourage you to go to their online dispensary where they have curated a spectrum of supplements that they have found effective for creating skin health and beauty.

If you ask this one question of your aesthetic provider, only to be greeted by some version of the following:
- "You just need to eat less and exercise more."
- "You get all the nutrients you need from the food you eat."
- "Supplements are worthless."
- "There's no connection between diet and your skin."

I would suggest that you very seriously consider moving on from receiving care from an aesthetic practitioner whose knowledge base fossilized decades early. At the very least, the professional should acknowledge your concern and direct you to a personalized nutrition practitioner who can address your questions and guide you in the right direction.

The Quest for Synergy

In the foreword to this book, Dr. Day pointed out my love of synergy, and how the whole can be greater than the sum of its parts. To this end, I'd like to introduce one more term—*integrative aesthetics*.

> *Integrative Aesthetics* encompasses personalized assessments, treatments, and counseling that recognize skin health and beauty as highly dependent upon multiple organ systems that are themselves affected by nutritional genomics, lifestyle, and environment.

Integrative aesthetics is my call to both sides of the aisle: the functional doctors who think of skin beauty as a privilege, and the aesthetic physicians who consider nutrition to be interesting but ultimately not important for their area of expertise. In my synergistic view of the world, I see these two disciplines coming together. I'm encouraged by the words of JD McCoy, ND. While trained as a naturopathic doctor, he now runs an aesthetic center (contourmedical.com) in Gilbert, AZ. Dr. McCoy points to the issues and opportunities facing practitioners today.

"What you learn really quickly is that patients are just not getting wellness and nutrition support from their traditional primary care provider. Many of my patients actually spend more time with me, doing cosmetic treatments, than they do to with any of their primary care providers. We'll talk about a lot of different things related to their health and wellbeing. I've been able to respond to this need by integrating more hormone optimization and diet recommendations into my cosmetic treatments. The same patients who are investing in looking good are the exact same patients who are willing to invest to feel good too. We're starting to see our patients younger. They're thinking preventively about the appearance of their skin. So, it's the perfect audience to talk about preventing disease."

A Few Final Thoughts

As someone who has traveled the world speaking and teaching (I've racked up more than 5 million actual miles on American Airlines alone), there's one phrase I master in every foreign country. The sounds are unique—*na zdarovya, kampei, salud, gambei*—but the words all translate into "cheers." This is a common shared experience. It begins with a moment of reflection, a meeting of the eyes, and a shared utterance; finally, it's topped off with the clink of glasses touching. Most often the toast is one of gratitude, praise, or wishes for a bright future. I hope you have had some moments in your reading when you too could behold a brighter future, one in which you gain the energy and vitality of optimal health, and the brilliant glow from your radiant skin. So, to you, I say, thank you for taking this time to be with me through the pages of my book, I wish you well, and cheers.

> **STAY IN TOUCH**
> Want more tips on skin health and beauty from inside out? Then stay in touch. I'll be periodically coming out with new content, a few videos, and some great learning opportunities.
> Visit me at drtager.com, by email at:
> contact@drtager.com
> IG @drmtager
> Healthcare Professionals: Join me on LinkedIn

For those who wish to purchase volume copies of *Feed Your Skin Right* for your organization, please send an email request to FYSR@changewell.com.

APPENDIX A

RDAS FOR SELECT VITAMINS & MINERALS IMPORTANT FOR SKIN HEALTH

VITAMINS

Biotin (Vitamin B7): Adults, Age 19+
- Men .... 30 mcg/day
- Women .... 30 mcg/day
- Pregnancy .... 30 mcg/day
- Lactation .... 35 mcg/day

Folate: Adults, Age 19+
- Men .... 400 mcg/day
- Women .... 400 mcg/day*
- Pregnancy .... 600 mcg/day
- Lactation .... 500 mcg/day

* Any woman planning to become pregnant (or is sexually active and not using birth control) should take folic acid at the pregnancy-recommended level.

Vitamin B6: Adults, Age 19+
- Men 19-50 .... 1.3 mg/day
- Men 50+ .... 1.7 mg/day
- Women 19-50 .... 1.3 mg/day
- Women 50+ .... 1.5 mg/day
- Pregnancy .... 1.9 mg/day
- Lactation .... 2.0 mg/day

Vitamin B12: Adults, Age 14+
- Men .... 2.4 mcg/day
- Women .... 2.4 mcg/day

- Pregnancy .... 2.6 mcg/day
- Lactation .... 2.8 mcg/day

Vitamin C: Adults, Age 19+
- Men .... 90 mg/day*
- Women .... 75 mg/day*

*Smokers of either gender require an additional 35 mg/day to attenuate oxidative damage caused by smoking.

Vitamin A: Adults, Age 19+
- Men .... 900 mcg RAE/day
- Women .... 700 mcg RAE/day
- Pregnancy .... 770 mcg RAE/day
- Lactation .... 1300 mcg RAE/day

The Food and Drug Administration (FDA) updated its requirements in January 2020 as to how vitamin A is listed on the Nutrition Facts and Supplement Facts labels. Previously, it was listed as international units (IUs); now it is mcg RAE (retinol activity equivalents). RAE depends on

---

CONVERSION BETWEEN INTERNATIONAL UNITS (IU) AND RETINOL ACTIVITY EQUIVALENTS (RAE)*

- 1 IU retinol = 0.3 mcg RAE
- 1 IU supplemental beta-carotene = 0.3 mcg RAE
- 1 IU dietary beta-carotene = 0.05 mcg RAE
- 1 IU dietary alpha-carotene or beta-cryptoxanthin = 0.025 mcg RAE

Conversion is only possible if the source(s) of vitamin A is known and mixed source diets can be challenging to calculate. An RDA of 900 mcg RAE equals:

- 3,000 IU if the food source is preformed vitamin A
- 3,000 IU if the supplement is preformed vitamin A
- 3,000 IU if the supplement is beta-carotene
- 18,000 IU if the food source is beta-carotene
- 36,000 IU if the food source is alpha-carotene or beta-cryptoxanthin

the source of vitamin A. One mcg RAE is equivalent to 1 mcg retinol, 2 mcg supplemental beta-carotene, 12 mcg dietary beta-carotene, or 24 mcg dietary alpha-carotene or beta-cryptoxanthin.[213] Manufacturer compliance was expected by January 2021.

Vitamin D$_3$: Adults, Age 19+
- Men 19-70 .... 15 mcg/day (600 IU)
- Men 70+ .... 20 mcg/day (800 IU)
- Women 19-70 .... 15 mcg/day (600 IU)
- Women 70+ .... 20 mcg/day (800 IU)
- Pregnancy .... 15 mcg/day (600 IU)
- Lactation .... 15 mcg/day (600 IU)

Vitamin E (Alpha-Tocopherol): Adults, Age 14+
- Men .... 15 mg/day
- Women .... 15 mg/day
- Pregnancy .... 15 mg/day
- Lactation .... 19 mg/day

As of January 2021, vitamin E must be listed on the new Nutrition Facts and Supplement Labels in milligrams (mg) instead of international units (IU).

CONVERSION BETWEEN INTERNATIONAL UNITS (IU) AND MILLIGRAMS (mg)

- 1 IU natural alpha-tocopherol (food) = 0.67mg
- 1 IU synthetic alpha-tocopherol (supplement) = 0.45mg

Vitamin K: Adults, Age 19+
- Men .... 120 mcg/day
- Women .... 90 mcg/day
- Pregnancy .... 90 mcg/day
- Lactation .... 90 mcg/day

MINERALS

Calcium: Adults, Age 19+
- Men 19-50 .... 1,000 mg/day
- Men 51-70 .... 1,000 mg/day
- Men 71+ .... 1,200 mg/day
- Women 19-50 .... 1,000 mg/day
- Women 51-70 .... 1,200 mg/day
- Women 71+ .... 1,200 mg/day
- Pregnancy .... 1,000 mg/day
- Lactation .... 1,000 mg/day

Copper: Adults, Age 19+
- Men .... 900 mcg/day
- Women .... 900 mcg/day
- Pregnancy .... 1300 mcg/day
- Lactation .... 1300 mcg/day

Magnesium: Adults, Age 19+
- Men 19-30 .... 400 mg/day
- Men 31+ .... 420 mg/day
- Women 19-30 .... 310 mg/day
- Women 31+ .... 320 mg/day
- Pregnancy 19-30 .... 350 mg/day
- Pregnancy 31+ .... 360 mg/day
- Lactation 19-30 .... 310 mg/day
- Lactation 31+ .... 320 mg/day

Potassium: Adults, Age 19+
- Men .... 3,400 mg/day
- Women .... 2,600 mg/day
- Pregnancy .... 2,900 mg/day
- Lactation .... 2,800 mg/day

Selenium: Adults, Age 19+
- Men .... 55 mcg/day
- Women .... 55 mcg/day
- Pregnancy .... 60 mcg/day
- Lactation .... 70 mcg/day

Zinc: Adults, Age 19+
- Men .... 11 mg/day
- Women .... 8 mg/day
- Pregnancy .... 11 mg/day
- Lactation .... 12 mg/day

APPENDIX B

MICRONUTRIENT DEFICIENCIES & EXCESSIVE INTAKES

Excessive Intake of BIOTIN

No tolerable upper intake level for biotin has been established because there is no evidence of toxicity when taken in large amounts—up to 200 mg/day. Remember: the RDA is in micrograms, not milligrams, so this is a large amount. The practical drawback to taking a lot of supplemental biotin—or just taking more than the RDA—is that it can result in skewed laboratory tests.[214] Falsely high or falsely low results may result in a misdiagnosis or inappropriate prescribed treatment. In the case of thyroid function tests, excessive biotin use can lead to an incorrect hyperthyroidism diagnosis or a misinterpretation that the thyroid hormone dose is too high.[215] If you take biotin supplements, you should discontinue taking it at least 2 days prior to your thyroid test.

FOLATE Deficiency

A dietary folate deficiency is rare, although possible, resulting in macrocytic (megaloblastic) anemia—a type of anemia characterized by unusually large red blood cells. Typically, a folate deficiency is caused by something else such as alcohol and certain medications (methotrexate, anticonvulsants, sulfa drugs) or GI conditions which may interfere with the body's ability to either absorb or utilize folate. Deficiencies of folate and vitamins B6 and B12 play a role in the accumulation of homocysteine in the blood, which increases cardiovascular disease risk. A folate deficiency may also be caused by a variant in the MTHFR gene, which hinders the conversion of dietary folate into its active form. (See a more detailed description under Vitamin B12.)

Excessive Intake of FOLATE

The tolerable upper intake level is 1000 mcg/day. Exceeding this could potentially mask a vitamin B12 deficiency, and some research suggests it may increase the risk of colon cancer in susceptible individuals.[216]

VITAMIN B6 Deficiency

A vitamin B6 "insufficiency" is probably the most accurate term when describing the types of Americans likely to be affected: patients with chronic and autoimmune diseases which impair absorption (celiac disease, Crohn's disease, inflammatory bowel disease, and ulcerative colitis).

Excessive Intake of VITAMIN B6

There is no evidence that eating too much vitamin B6 from foods has any adverse effects. The FDA's tolerable upper intake level is 100 mg/day, which is about 60 times more than the RDA. It would be quite difficult to achieve the upper limit from foods alone.

VITAMIN B12 Deficiency

Vitamin B12 deficiency is fairly common in the U.S. general population, affecting between 1.5% and 15%.[217] It is also more common after age 40.[218] The cause of a person's deficiency is often unknown, but certain situations increase the risk, including pernicious anemia, insufficient absorption from food—either post-surgery or in general—dietary deficiency (vegetarian/vegan lifestyle), and taking medications that reduce the output of hydrochloric acid in the stomach (Prilosec,® Prevacid,® Tagamet,® Pepcid,® and Zantac®). Symptoms of vitamin B12 deficiency include macrocytic anemia, fatigue, weakness, lack of appetite, constipation, weight loss, and elevated blood levels of homocysteine.

Neurological symptoms include numbness or tingling in the feet or hands, balance problems, depression, poor memory, confusion, and cognitive impairment; a vitamin B12 deficiency is commonly mistaken for the onset of dementia in older persons.

Excessive Intake of VITAMIN B12

There is no tolerable upper intake level for vitamin B12 since it has a very low risk of toxicity.

Excessive Intake of VITAMIN C

Taking more than 2000mg/day can cause GI upset due to the acidity. High intakes may increase the risk of calcium oxalate kidney stones in susceptible individuals. If you want to take more than the upper limit for immune support, it's a good idea to spread out the vitamin C over the course of the day and/or take a buffered form.

VITAMIN A Deficiency
Vitamin A deficiency (VAD) is very rare among Americans unless the BCO1 gene variant is present. This may be compounded by veganism.

Excessive Intake of VITAMIN A (Hypervitaminosis A)
Taking too much preformed vitamin A can be toxic, causing hypervitaminosis A. The tolerable upper intake level for adults 19 and older is 3000mcg/day. Generally, hypervitaminosis A occurs from long-term supplement use—not food intake—and can result in a variety of symptoms including dizziness, headaches, nausea, joint or bone pain, skin rashes, coma, or death. Even if discontinued, build-up in the liver dissipates slowly and damage may be irreversible. Taking large quantities of provitamin A carotenoids does not have the same effect.

Excessive Intake of VITAMIN D
Taking too much vitamin D from supplements can be toxic because it increases the amount of calcium that is absorbed through the small intestine. For people who want to supplement vitamin D at levels greater than the tolerable upper intake level of 4,000 IU a day, testing your vitamin D level before and during treatment is important.

VITAMIN E Deficiency
Deficiency is rare and does not produce any discernable symptoms in healthy people. Patients with fat-malabsorption disorders are susceptible to a deficiency because vitamin E must be absorbed along with a fat. In this case, symptoms include peripheral neuropathy, retinopathy, muscle weakness and atrophy, loss of muscle control, or impaired immune function.

Excessive Intake of VITAMIN E
There is no risk of consuming excess vitamin E from natural food sources. Limited human studies suggest, however, that high-dose (greater than 400 IU/day [180mg/day]) synthetic alpha-tocopherol may increase the risk of death from any cause and should be avoided.[219] The FDA's tolerable upper intake level is 1,000 mg/day for natural alpha-tocopherol and 1,100mg/day for the synthetic version was established based on the possible risk of supplemental vitamin E causing unwanted bleeding (hemorrhage). There are no limits established for tocotrienols.

VITAMIN K Deficiency

Deficiency in adults eating a varied diet is extremely rare because vitamin K is found in many commonly-eaten foods. Patients who have malabsorption disorders, GI diseases (celiac disease, short bowel syndrome, ulcerative colitis), or underwent gastric bypass surgery can develop a deficiency.

Excessive Intake of VITAMIN K

Due to the low risk of toxicity, no tolerable upper intake level for vitamin K has been established.

CALCIUM Deficiency (Hypocalcemia)

Because calcium levels in the blood are so tightly regulated, a short-term insufficient dietary intake will not produce any discernable symptoms. Osteopenia (weak bones) and osteoporosis (brittle bones) are more common with long-term inadequate calcium intake in otherwise healthy individuals. Calcium inadequacy is more likely in post-menopausal women, vegetarians, vegans, and individuals with lactose intolerance.

Excessive Intake of CALCIUM (Hypercalcemia)

Again, because the body's blood calcium levels are so tightly regulated, excessively high levels in the blood (hypercalcemia) are generally the result of a malignancy, abnormal parathyroid hormone levels (hyperparathyroidism), or possibly, over-supplementation. This leads to compromised kidney function, elevated calcium levels in the urine, kidney stones, constipation, and calcification of vascular tissue (hardening of the arteries). The tolerable upper intake level for adults ages 19-50 is 2,500 mg/day, and for ages 71 and older, is 2,000 mg/day.

COPPER Deficiency

Although uncommon, a copper deficiency can result in anemia, elevated cholesterol levels, low skin pigmentation (hypopigmentation), osteoporosis, connective tissue disorders, lack of muscle control or coordination, and increased infection risk. Copper inadequacy is more prevalent in patients who have celiac disease or Menkes disease, the result of a rare genetic variant in the *ATP7A* gene. Taking megadose quantities of zinc supplements can interfere with copper absorption.

Excessive Intake of COPPER
Copper toxicity is relative rare except in the case of Wilson's disease, a variant in the *ATP7B* gene, which leads to a build-up of copper in the tissues. Excessive exposure from copper that has leached from the water pipes supplying tap water can also be problematic. Chronic, high-level exposure causes GI symptoms such as abdominal pain, cramping, nausea, vomiting, diarrhea, and liver damage. The tolerable upper intake level for copper is 10,000 mcg/day.

MAGNESIUM Deficiency (Hypomagnesaemia)
Even if a healthy individual does not consume sufficient dietary magnesium, the kidneys will hold on to as much as they can to avoid a deficiency. Magnesium intake for all Americans—and Western societies—regardless of age, is falling short of the RDA and it's commonly showing up on routine bloodwork. Many physicians are now recommending supplementation.

Excessive Intake of MAGNESIUM
Obtaining too much magnesium from food is nearly impossible in healthy people because their kidneys eliminate whatever the body doesn't need. Supplemental magnesium or magnesium-containing medications in large doses (greater than 5,000 mg/day) may result in nausea, abdominal cramps, and diarrhea. This occurs because the magnesium stays in the GI tract and stimulates gastric motility rather than being absorbed. Laxative effects are associated with 4 types of magnesium—magnesium carbonate, chloride, gluconate, and oxide.[220] There is no tolerable upper intake level for dietary magnesium, but the FDA recommends adults take no more than 350 mg/day of supplemental magnesium.

POTASSIUM Deficiency (Hypokalemia)
In general, Americans' potassium consumption is lower than recommended, probably because of low quantities of fruits and vegetables in the diet. Thus, potassium has been designated as a "nutrient of public health concern."[221] People who don't get enough potassium in their diets experience increased blood pressure, salt sensitivity (sodium can dramatically increase blood pressure), increased excretion of calcium, more bone tissue degradation, and elevated risk of kidney stones.

A magnesium deficiency can contribute to hypokalemia by causing the kidneys to excrete potassium. Potassium inadequacy is common in patients who have inflammatory bowel disease or chronic diarrhea. Diuretics and laxatives also increase potassium excretion.

Excessive Intake of POTASSIUM (Hyperkalemia)
A high dietary potassium intake does not pose any known health risks in people with normal kidney function because the kidneys will excrete what the body doesn't need in the urine. Thus, there is no tolerable upper intake level for potassium in otherwise healthy people. Patients who have compromised kidney function or take certain hypertension medications can develop hyperkalemia. Severe cases present with muscle weakness, paralysis, rapid heartbeat, or life-threatening abnormal heart rhythms.

SELENIUM Deficiency
Americans in general do not suffer from selenium deficiency; people living in the West and Midwest tend to have higher stored selenium levels than people living in South and Northeast.[222] Lower levels of selenium have been reported in people who consume foods grown in low-selenium soil, kidney dialysis patients, and people living with HIV. Male infertility is more prevalent in men with a selenium deficiency.

Excessive Intake of SELENIUM (Selenosis)
Getting too much selenium over a long period of time—either from foods or supplements—can result in hair and nail brittleness or loss, a condition attributed to selenosis. The FDA's tolerable upper intake level for selenium (400 mcg/day) is based on the amount that induces hair and nail issues. An early sign is having garlic breath (without eating garlic) and a metallic taste in the mouth.

ZINC Deficiency
Although zinc deficiency is relatively rare in the United States, older adults may have less-than-optimal intakes due to food insufficiency. Zinc-absorption problems are common with digestive diseases, vegetarianism or veganism, alcoholism, and sickle cell anemia.

Excessive Intake of ZINC

Zinc toxicity can result from acute or chronic consumption of high dose supplements. Headaches, loss of appetite, nausea, vomiting, abdominal cramps, and diarrhea can occur relatively soon after ingestion. Chronic supplementation with doses in the range of 150-450 mg/day can inhibit copper absorption, interfere with iron function, decrease good (HDL) cholesterol, and lower immune function. Because zinc supplements often interact with common medications and other supplements, your physician can recommend ideal spacing between them. The tolerable upper limit intake for zinc is 40mg/day.

APPENDIX C

COMMON GENETIC VARIANTS & SKIN HEALTH*

Gene	Contribution	SNP Variation or Gene Form	Beneficial Nutrients[223]
APOA5	Vitamin E deficiency	SNPs reduce the amount of circulating vitamin E.	Vitamin E
BCO1	Vitamin A deficiency	SNPs prevent conversion of beta-carotene into retinal, a usable form of vitamin A which is necessary for cell membrane and skin protection.	Vitamin A (beta-carotene)
CYP2R1	Vitamin D deficiency	SNPs reduce the amount of circulating vitamin D3.	Vitamin D Iron Calcium
GC	Vitamin D deficiency	SNPs reduce the amount of circulating vitamin D3.	Vitamin D Calcium
GSTT1	Vitamin C deficiency	Gene exists in either insertion or deletion form; deletion form results in a decreased ability to process vitamin C from the diet.	Vitamin C
IRF4	Solar brown spots Seborrheic keratosis (non-cancer, waxy, scaly raised lesions with age)	SNPs may translate cumulative UV exposure into pigmentation spots.	
GLO1	Loss of elasticity Fine lines and wrinkles	SNPs reduce capacity for AGEs to be neutralized, leading to fragility of collagen and elastin in the skin.	

Gene	Effects	Mechanism	Nutrients
MC1R	Skin pigmentation Increased risk of photoaging Increased risk of melanoma	SNPs control the type of melanin (pheomelanin and eumelanin) and amount of expressed in the melanocytes.	
MMP1	Loss of elasticity Skin inflammation Increased risk of photoaging	SNPs causes increased rates of collagenase production which accelerates the breakdown of collagen in the skin.	
MTHFR	Folate deficiency Skin pigmentation Increased risk of vitiligo & plaque psoriasis	SNPs impair capacity to metabolize dietary folate and folic acid which is necessary for other products vital to the synthesis of DNA, RNA and amino acids.	Vitamin B2 Folate Vitamin B6 Vitamin B12 Magnesium
NQO1	Premature aging Loss of antioxidant capacity	SNPs leads to a build-up of the superoxide radicals, a type of free radical which damages skin.	Vitamin B2 Glutathione
SLC30A3	Zinc inadequacy	SNPs reduce the amount of circulating zinc.	Zinc
SOD2	Premature aging Loss of antioxidant capacity	SNPs leads to a build-up of the superoxide radicals, a type of free radical which damages skin.	Manganese Vitamin C Vitamin E Vitamin A Curcumin Zeaxanthin Lutein

* Courtesy of Nutrigenomix

> For more information about human genes, their normal functions, and how genetic variants affect your health, visit the National Library of Medicine's GENES webpage at https://medlineplus.gov/genetics/gene.

BIBLIOGRAPHY

[1] Paoli, Antonio et al. "The Influence of Meal Frequency and Timing on Health in Humans: The Role of Fasting." *Nutrients* vol. 11,4 719. 28 Mar. 2019.

[2] Patterson, Ruth E, and Dorothy D Sears. "Metabolic Effects of Intermittent Fasting." *Annual review of nutrition* vol. 37 (2017): 371-393.

[3] "Dirty Dozen™ EWG's 2021 Shopper's Guide to Pesticides in Produce™." *Environmental Working Group*, www.ewg.org/foodnews/dirty-dozen.php.

[4] "The Toxic Twelve Chemicals and Contaminants in Cosmetics." *Environmental Working Group*, 5 May 2020, www.ewg.org/the-toxic-twelve-chemicals-and-contaminants-in-cosmetics.

[5] Adams, Kelly M et al. "Nutrition education in U.S. medical schools: latest update of a national survey." *Academic medicine: journal of the Association of American Medical Colleges* vol. 85,9 (2010): 1537-42.

[6] Yanez, JoAnn, et al. "What Advanced Nutrition Training Do Naturopathic Doctors Receive?" *Institute for Natural Medicine*, naturemed.org/faq/faq-what-advanced-nutrition-training-do-naturopathic-doctors-receive.

[7] "Dietary Supplement Use Among Adults: United States, 2017–2018." *Centers for Disease Control and Prevention*, Feb. 2021, www.cdc.gov/nchs/products/databriefs/db399.htm#section_3.

[8] "10 Positive Steps to Immune Resilience." *American Nutrition Association*, theana.org/Immuneresilience/ANAPublicResources/10steps.

[9] "Boosting Immunity: Functional Medicine Tips on Prevention & Optimizing Immune Function During the COVID-19 (Coronavirus) Outbreak." *Institute for Functional Medicine*, www.ifm.org/news-insights/boosting-immunity-functional-medicine-tips-prevention-immunity-boosting-covid-19-coronavirus-outbreak.

[10] "The Functional Medicine Approach to COVID-19: Virus-Specific Nutraceutical and Botanical Agents." *Institute for Functional Medicine*, 15 Oct. 2021, www.ifm.org/news-insights/the-functional-medicine-approach-to-covid-19-virus-specific-nutraceutical-and-botanical-agents.

[11] Morton, Claire. "The Analyst's Take: Is 'Beauty From Within' the Trend to Watch?" *New Hope Network*, 14 Oct. 2021, www.newhope.com/market-data-and-analysis/analysts-take-beauty-within-trend-watch.

[12] "Obesity Is a Common, Serious, and Costly Disease." *Centers for Disease Control and Prevention*, 12 Nov. 2021, www.cdc.gov/obesity/data/adult.html.

[13] "Facts About Hypertension | cdc.gov." *Centers for Disease Control and Prevention*, 27 Sept. 2021, www.cdc.gov/bloodpressure/facts.htm.

[14] "National Diabetes Statistics Report, 2020 | CDC." *Centers for Disease Control and Prevention*, www.cdc.gov/diabetes/data/statistics-report/index.html. Accessed 28 Dec. 2021.

[15] Ferdman, Roberto. "Where People around the World Eat the Most Sugar and Fat." *Washington Post*, 5 Feb. 2015, www.washingtonpost.com/news/wonk/wp/2015/02/05/where-people-around-the-world-eat-the-most-sugar-and-fat.

[16] Pariona, Amber. "Countries That Eat the Most Sugar." *WorldAtlas*, 18 Mar. 2019, www.worldatlas.com/articles/top-sugar-consuming-nations-in-the-world.html.

[17] DeSilver, Drew. "What's on Your Table? How America's Diet Has Changed over the Decades." *Pew Research Center*, 13 Dec. 2016, www.pewresearch.org/fact-tank/2016/12/13/whats-on-your-table-how-americas-diet-has-changed-over-the-decades.

[18] Gkogkolou, Paraskevi, and Markus Böhm. "Advanced glycation end products: Key players in skin aging?." *Dermato-endocrinology* vol. 4,3 (2012): 259-70.

[19] Helander, Marjo et al. "Glyphosate decreases mycorrhizal colonization and affects plant-soil feedback." *The Science of the total environment* vol. 642 (2018): 285-291.

[20] Chassaing, Benoit et al. "Dietary emulsifiers impact the mouse gut microbiota promoting colitis and metabolic syndrome." *Nature* vol. 519,7541 (2015): 92-6.

[21] Chassaing, Benoit et al. "Dietary emulsifiers directly alter human microbiota composition and gene expression ex vivo potentiating intestinal inflammation." *Gut* vol. 66,8 (2017): 1414-1427.

[22] Bancil, Aaron S et al. "Food additive emulsifiers and their impact on gut microbiome, permeability and inflammation: mechanistic insights in inflammatory bowel disease." *Journal of Crohn's & colitis*, jjaa254. 18 Dec. 2020.

[23] Viennois, Emilie et al. "Dietary Emulsifier-Induced Low-Grade Inflammation Promotes Colon Carcinogenesis." *Cancer research* vol. 77,1 (2017): 27-40.

[24] Suez, Jotham et al. "Artificial sweeteners induce glucose intolerance by altering the gut microbiota." *Nature* vol. 514,7521 (2014): 181-6.

[25] *Innovative Healing Academy*. www.innovativehealingacademy.com. Accessed 28 Dec. 2021.

[26] Igbinedion, Samuel O et al. "Non-celiac gluten sensitivity: All wheat attack is not celiac." *World journal of gastroenterology* vol. 23,40 (2017): 7201-7210.

[27] Gallup, Inc., and Rebecca Riffkin. "One in Five Americans Include Gluten-Free Foods in Diet." *Gallup.Com*, 22 May 2021, news.gallup.com/poll/184307/one-five-americans-include-gluten-free-foods-diet.aspx.

[28] Skodje, Gry I et al. "Fructan, Rather Than Gluten, Induces Symptoms in Patients With Self-Reported Non-Celiac Gluten Sensitivity." *Gastroenterology* vol. 154,3 (2018): 529-539.e2.

[29] Koster, Maranke I. "Making an epidermis." *Annals of the New York Academy of Sciences* vol. 1170 (2009): 7-10.

[30] Fatima, Rawish, and Muhammad Aziz. "Achlorhydria." *NCBI Bookshelf*, 25 July 2017, www.ncbi.nlm.nih.gov/books/NBK507793/.

[31] Volpi, Elena et al. "Muscle tissue changes with aging." *Current opinion in clinical nutrition and metabolic care* vol. 7,4 (2004): 405-10.

[32] Agrimag. "Children Should Be Taught How to Grow Food in School and Here's Why." *Agriculture Monthly*, 3 June 2019, www.agriculture.com.ph/2019/06/12/children-should-be-taught-how-to-grow-food-in-school-and-heres-why.

[33] "DirtyDozen Fruits and Vegetables with the Most Pesticides – @EWG's Shopper's Guide to Pesticides in Produce™." *Environmental Working Group*, www.ewg.org/foodnews/dirty-dozen.php. Accessed 28 Dec. 2021.

[34] Emiroğlu, Nazan et al. "Insulin resistance in severe acne vulgaris." *Postepy dermatologii i alergologii* vol. 32,4 (2015): 281-5.

[35] Greenberg, Sophie A. "Diet and skin: a primer." *Cutis* vol. 106,5 (2020): E31-E32.

[36] Thomsen, Bryce J et al. "The Potential Uses of Omega-3 Fatty Acids in Dermatology: A Review." *Journal of cutaneous medicine and surgery* vol. 24,5 (2020): 481-494.

[37] Polcz, Monica E, and Adrian Barbul. "The Role of Vitamin A in Wound Healing." *Nutrition in clinical practice : official publication of the American Society for Parenteral and Enteral Nutrition* vol. 34,5 (2019): 695-700.

[38] LaRosa, Caroline L et al. "Consumption of dairy in teenagers with and without acne." *Journal of the American Academy of Dermatology* vol. 75,2 (2016): 318-22.

[39] Ramírez-Sánchez, Israel et al. "(-)-Epicatechin-induced recovery of mitochondria from simulated diabetes: Potential role of endothelial nitric oxide synthase." Diabetes & vascular disease research vol. 13,3 (2016): 201-10.

[40] Faccinetto-Beltrán, Paulinna et al. "Chocolate as Carrier to Deliver Bioactive Ingredients: Current Advances and Future Perspectives." Foods (Basel, Switzerland) vol. 10,9 2065. 1 Sep. 2021.

[41] Rynders, Corey A et al. "Effectiveness of Intermittent Fasting and Time-Restricted Feeding Compared to Continuous Energy Restriction for Weight Loss." *Nutrients* vol. 11,10 2442. 14 Oct. 2019.

[42] "CDC - How Much Sleep Do I Need? - Sleep and Sleep Disorders." *Centers for Disease Control and Prevention*, www.cdc.gov/sleep/about_sleep/how_much_sleep.html. Accessed 28 Dec. 2021.

[43] "KetoFLEX 12/3." *Apollo Health*, 17 Nov. 2021, www.apollohealthco.com/ketoflex-12-3.

[44] Pijl, Hanno. "Longevity. The allostatic load of dietary restriction." *Physiology & behavior* vol. 106,1 (2012): 51-7.

[45] Hwangbo, Dae-Sung et al. "Mechanisms of Lifespan Regulation by Calorie Restriction and Intermittent Fasting in Model Organisms." *Nutrients* vol. 12,4 1194. 24 Apr. 2020.

[46] Choi, Yeon Ja. "Shedding Light on the Effects of Calorie Restriction and its Mimetics on Skin Biology." *Nutrients* vol. 12,5 1529. 24 May. 2020.

[47] Luo, Ming-Jie et al. "Fasting before or after wound injury accelerates wound healing through the activation of pro-angiogenic SMOC1 and SCG2." *Theranostics* vol. 10,8 3779-3792. 19 Feb. 2020.

[48] Institute of Medicine (US) Committee on Quality of Health Care in America. *Crossing the Quality Chasm: A New Health System for the 21st Century*. National Academies Press (US), 2001.

[49] Nestor, Mark S et al. "Safety and Efficacy of Oral Polypodium leucotomos Extract in Healthy Adult Subjects." *The Journal of clinical and aesthetic dermatology* vol. 8,2 (2015): 19-23.

[50] Truzzi, Francesca et al. "An Overview on Dietary Polyphenols and Their Biopharmaceutical Classification System (BCS)." *International journal of molecular sciences* vol. 22,11 5514. 24 May. 2021.

[51] "Fruits and Vegetables Serving Sizes Infographic." *American Heart Association*, 2017, www.heart.org/en/healthy-living/healthy-eating/add-color/fruits-and-vegetables-serving-sizes.

[52] Poyet, M et al. "A library of human gut bacterial isolates paired with longitudinal multiomics data enables mechanistic microbiome research." *Nature medicine* vol. 25,9 (2019): 1442-1452.

[53] Tan, Jian et al. "The role of short-chain fatty acids in health and disease." *Advances in immunology* vol. 121 (2014): 91-119.

[54] Reichardt, Nicole et al. "Phylogenetic distribution of three pathways for propionate production within the human gut microbiota." *The ISME journal* vol. 8,6 (2014): 1323-35.

[55] Dalile, Boushra et al. "The role of short-chain fatty acids in microbiota-gut-brain communication." *Nature reviews. Gastroenterology & hepatology* vol. 16,8 (2019): 461-478.

[56] Schwarz, Agatha et al. "The Short-Chain Fatty Acid Sodium Butyrate Functions as a Regulator of the Skin Immune System." *The Journal of investigative dermatology* vol. 137,4 (2017): 855-864.

[57] McDonald, Lawrence Clifford. "Effects of short- and long-course antibiotics on the lower intestinal microbiome as they relate to traveller's diarrhea." *Journal of travel medicine* vol. 24,suppl_1 (2017): S35-S38.

[58] Vich Vila, Arnau et al. "Impact of commonly used drugs on the composition and metabolic function of the gut microbiota." *Nature communications* vol. 11,1 362. 17 Jan. 2020.

[59] Bailey, M. T., Dowd, S. E., Galley, J. D., Hufnagle, A. R., Allen, R. G., & Lyte, M. (2011). Exposure to a social stressor alters the structure of the intestinal microbiota: implications for stressor-induced immunomodulation. *Brain, behavior, and immunity, 25*(3), 397–407.

[60] Fasano, Alessio. "Zonulin and its regulation of intestinal barrier function: the biological door to inflammation, autoimmunity, and cancer." *Physiological reviews* vol. 91,1 (2011): 151-75.

[61] Odenwald, Matthew A, and Jerrold R Turner. "Intestinal permeability defects: is it time to treat?." *Clinical gastroenterology and hepatology: the official clinical practice journal of the American Gastroenterological Association* vol. 11,9 (2013): 1075-83.

[62] Sikora, Mariusz et al. "Clinical Implications of Intestinal Barrier Damage in Psoriasis." *Journal of inflammation research* vol. 14 237-243. 27 Jan. 2021.

[63] Drago, L et al. "Probiotics: immunomodulatory properties in allergy and eczema." *Giornale italiano di dermatologia e venereologia : organo ufficiale, Societa italiana di dermatologia e sifilografia* vol. 148,5 (2013): 505-14.

[64] Fedrigo, Aiessa et al. "ASCA (Anti-Saccharomyces cerevisiae Antibody) in Patients With Scleroderma." *Journal of clinical rheumatology: practical reports on rheumatic & musculoskeletal diseases* vol. 25,1 (2019): 24-27.

[65] Vich Vila, Arnau et al. "Impact of commonly used drugs on the composition and metabolic function of the gut microbiota." *Nature communications* vol. 11,1 362. 17 Jan. 2020.

[66] Playford, Raymond John, and Michael James Weiser. "Bovine Colostrum: Its Constituents and Uses." *Nutrients* vol. 13,1 265. 18 Jan. 2021.

[67] Playford, R J et al. "Bovine colostrum is a health food supplement which prevents NSAID induced gut damage." *Gut* vol. 44,5 (1999): 653-8.

[68] Pugh, Jamie N et al. "Glutamine supplementation reduces markers of intestinal permeability during running in the heat in a dose-dependent manner." *European journal of applied physiology* vol. 117,12 (2017): 2569-2577.

[69] Shariatpanahi, Zahra Vahdat et al. "Effects of Early Enteral Glutamine Supplementation on Intestinal Permeability in Critically Ill Patients." *Indian journal of critical care medicine: peer-reviewed, official publication of Indian Society of Critical Care Medicine* vol. 23,8 (2019): 356-362.

[70] Davison, Glen et al. "Zinc carnosine works with bovine colostrum in truncating heavy exercise-induced increase in gut permeability in healthy volunteers." *The American journal of clinical nutrition* vol. 104,2 (2016): 526-36.

[71] Yu, Y et al. "Changing our microbiome: probiotics in dermatology." *The British journal of dermatology* vol. 182,1 (2020): 39-46.

[72] Kim, Dakyung et al. "Combination of *Bifidobacterium longum* and Galacto-Oligosaccharide Protects the Skin from Photoaging." *Journal of medicinal food* vol. 24,6 (2021): 606-616.

[73] Lee, Kippeum et al. "Exopolysaccharide from *Lactobacillus plantarum* HY7714 Protects against Skin Aging through Skin-Gut Axis Communication." *Molecules (Basel, Switzerland)* vol. 26,6 1651. 16 Mar. 2021.

[74] "Skin Care Products Market Size Report, 2021–2028." *Grand View Research*, Oct. 2021, www.grandviewresearch.com/industry-analysis/skin-care-products-market.

[75] Grice, Elizabeth A et al. "A diversity profile of the human skin microbiota." *Genome research* vol. 18,7 (2008): 1043-50.

[76] Grice, Elizabeth A, and Julia A Segre. "The skin microbiome." *Nature reviews. Microbiology* vol. 9,4 (2011): 244-53.

[77] Fitz-Gibbon, Sorel et al. "Propionibacterium acnes strain populations in the human skin microbiome associated with acne." *The Journal of investigative dermatology* vol. 133,9 (2013): 2152-60.

[78] "People at Genetic Risk for Alzheimer's Disease to Test Prevention Drugs." *National Institute on Aging*, 23 Aug. 2016, www.nia.nih.gov/news/people-genetic-risk-alzheimers-disease-test-prevention-drugs.

[79] "Genetic Testing." *NIH Medline Plus*, medlineplus.gov/download/genetics/understanding/testing.pdf. Accessed 28 Dec. 2021.

[80] Elfakir, Anissa et al. "Functional MC1R-gene variants are associated with increased risk for severe photoaging of facial skin." *The Journal of investigative dermatology* vol. 130,4 (2010): 1107-15.

[81] Jacobs, Leonie C et al. "A Genome-Wide Association Study Identifies the Skin Color Genes IRF4, MC1R, ASIP, and BNC2 Influencing Facial Pigmented Spots." *The Journal of investigative dermatology* vol. 135,7 (2015): 1735-1742.

[82] Praetorius, Christian et al. "A polymorphism in IRF4 affects human pigmentation through a tyrosinase-dependent MITF/TFAP2A pathway." *Cell* vol. 155,5 (2013): 1022-33.

[83] Bagheri Hamidi, Arash et al. "Association of MTHFR C677T polymorphism with elevated homocysteine level and disease development in vitiligo." *International journal of immunogenetics* vol. 47,4 (2020): 342-350.

[84] Karabacak, Ercan et al. "Methylenetetrahydrofolate reductase (MTHFR) 677C>T gene polymorphism as a possible factor for reducing clinical severity of psoriasis." *International journal of clinical and experimental medicine* vol. 7,3 697-702. 15 Mar. 2014.

[85] Iyer, Smita S et al. "Cysteine redox potential determines pro-inflammatory IL-1beta levels." *PloS one* vol. 4,3 (2009): e5017.

[86] Holick, Michael F, and Tai C Chen. "Vitamin D deficiency: a worldwide problem with health consequences." *The American journal of clinical nutrition* vol. 87,4 (2008): 1080S-6S.

[87] Ornish, Dean et al. "Changes in prostate gene expression in men undergoing an intensive nutrition and lifestyle intervention." *Proceedings of the National Academy of Sciences of the United States of America* vol. 105,24 (2008): 8369-74.

[88] Boroni, Mariana et al. "Highly accurate skin-specific methylome analysis algorithm as a platform to screen and validate therapeutics for healthy aging." *Clinical epigenetics* vol. 12,1 105. 13 Jul. 2020.

[89] Olesen, Caroline Meyer et al. "Advancement through epidermis using tape stripping technique and Reflectance Confocal Microscopy." *Scientific reports* vol. 9,1 12217. 21 Aug. 2019.

[90] Cintron, Dahima et al. "Effects of oral versus transdermal menopausal hormone treatments on self-reported sleep domains and their association with vasomotor symptoms in recently menopausal women enrolled in the Kronos Early Estrogen Prevention Study (KEEPS)." *Menopause (New York, N.Y.)* vol. 25,2 (2018): 145-153.

[91] Martin, Kathryn and Barbieri, Robert. Treatment of menopausal symptoms with hormone therapy. UpToDate. Waltham, MA: UpToDate Inc. https://www.uptodate.com/contents/treatment-of-menopausal-symptoms-with-hormone-therapy. Accessed on November 3, 2021.

[92] Glaser, Rebecca, and Constantine Dimitrakakis. "Testosterone therapy in women: myths and misconceptions." *Maturitas* vol. 74,3 (2013): 230-4.

[93] Smith, R N, and J W Studd. "Recent advances in hormone replacement therapy." *British journal of hospital medicine* vol. 49,11 (1993): 799-808.

[94] Papadakis, Georgios E et al. "Menopausal Hormone Therapy Is Associated With Reduced Total and Visceral Adiposity: The OsteoLaus Cohort." *The Journal of clinical endocrinology and metabolism* vol. 103,5 (2018): 1948-1957.

[95] Hellsten, Y and Gliemann, L. Limb vascular function in women: Effects of female sex hormones and physical therapy. *Transl Sports Medicine* 1 (2017): 14-24.

[96] Martin, Kathryn and Barbieri, Robert. Treatment of menopausal symptoms with hormone therapy. UpToDate. Waltham, MA: UpToDate Inc. https://www.uptodate.com/contents/treatment-of-menopausal-symptoms-with-hormone-therapy. Accessed 3 Nov. 2021.

[97] Yee, Brittany E et al. "Serum zinc levels and efficacy of zinc treatment in acne vulgaris: A systematic review and meta-analysis." *Dermatologic therapy* vol. 33,6 (2020): e14252.

[98] Cervantes, Jessica et al. "Effectiveness of Platelet-Rich Plasma for Androgenetic Alopecia: A Review of the Literature." *Skin appendage disorders* vol. 4,1 (2018): 1-11.

[99] Ablon, Glynis, and Steven Dayan. "A Randomized, Double-blind, Placebo-controlled, Multi-center, Extension Trial Evaluating the Efficacy of a New Oral Supplement in Women with Self-perceived Thinning Hair." *The Journal of clinical and aesthetic dermatology* vol. 8,12 (2015): 15-21.

[100] Stout, Roisin, and Mark Birch-Machin. "Mitochondria's Role in Skin Ageing." *Biology* vol. 8,2 29. 11 May. 2019.

[101] Krutmann, Jean, and Peter Schroeder. "Role of mitochondria in photoaging of human skin: the defective powerhouse model." *The journal of investigative dermatology. Symposium proceedings* vol. 14,1 (2009): 44-9.

[102] "Office of Dietary Supplements - Dietary Supplements for Primary Mitochondrial Disorders." *NIH Office of Dietary Supplements*, ods.od.nih.gov/factsheets/PrimaryMitochondrialDisorders-HealthProfessional. Accessed 28 Dec. 2021.

[103] Crane, J. D., MacNeil, L. G., Lally, J. S., Ford, R. J., Bujak, A. L., Brar, I. K., Kemp, B. E., Raha, S., Steinberg, G. R., & Tarnopolsky, M. A. (2015). Exercise-stimulated

interleukin-15 is controlled by AMPK and regulates skin metabolism and aging. *Aging cell*, *14*(4), 625–634.

[104] Couppé, Christian et al. "Life-long endurance running is associated with reduced glycation and mechanical stress in connective tissue." *Age (Dordrecht, Netherlands)* vol. 36,4 (2014): 9665.

[105] Richard, Michael J et al. "Analysis of the anatomic changes of the aging facial skeleton using computer-assisted tomography." *Ophthalmic plastic and reconstructive surgery* vol. 25,5 (2009): 382-6.

[106] Mendelson, B., & Wong, C. H. (2012). Changes in the facial skeleton with aging: implications and clinical applications in facial rejuvenation. *Aesthetic plastic surgery*, *36*(4), 753–760.

[107] McKendry, James et al. "Nutritional Supplements to Support Resistance Exercise in Countering the Sarcopenia of Aging." *Nutrients* vol. 12,7 2057. 10 Jul. 2020.

[108] Monda, V., Villano, I., Messina, A., Valenzano, A., Esposito, T., Moscatelli, F., Viggiano, A., Cibelli, G., Chieffi, S., Monda, M., & Messina, G. (2017). Exercise Modifies the Gut Microbiota with Positive Health Effects. *Oxidative medicine and cellular longevity*, *2017*, 3831972.

[109] Ribeiro, F. M., Petriz, B., Marques, G., Kamilla, L. H., & Franco, O. L. (2021). Is There an Exercise-Intensity Threshold Capable of Avoiding the Leaky Gut?. *Frontiers in nutrition*, *8*, 627289.

[110] Chan, Carmen W H et al. "The Association between Maternal Stress and Childhood Eczema: A Systematic Review." *International journal of environmental research and public health* vol. 15,3 395. 25 Feb. 2018.

[111] McCraty, Rollin, and Maria Zayas. "Intuitive Intelligence, Self-regulation, and Lifting Consciousness." *Global advances in health and medicine* vol. 3,2 (2014): 56-65.

[112] Wrede, Joanna E et al. "Mitochondrial DNA Copy Number in Sleep Duration Discordant Monozygotic Twins." *Sleep* vol. 38,10 1655-8. 1 Oct. 2015.

[113] Melhuish Beaupre, Lindsay M et al. "Mitochondria's role in sleep: Novel insights from sleep deprivation and restriction studies." *The world journal of biological psychiatry : the official journal of the World Federation of Societies of Biological Psychiatry*, 1-13. 6 May. 2021.

[114] "Physical Activity Guidelines for Americans - 2nd Edition." *U.S. Department of Health and Human Services*, health.gov/sites/default/files/2019-10/PAG_ExecutiveSummary.pdf. Accessed 28 Dec. 2021.

[115] "Tips for Exercising Without Flare-Ups | rosacea.org." *National Rosacea Society*, www.rosacea.org/rosacea-review/2007/summer/tips-for-exercising-without-flare-ups. Accessed 28 Dec. 2021.

[116] "Psoriasis Diet: Foods That Help Fight Inflammation." *Psoriasis Speaks*, www.psoriasis.com/living-with-psoriasis/psoriasis-diet-exercise?cid=ppc_ppd_mfst_psoriasis_de_exercise_and_psoriasis_phrase_US-IMMD-

200300&gclid=ea551cd6b9f519f07b5c7cb502a64b55&gclsrc=3p.ds&msclkid=ea551cd6b 9f519f07b5c7cb502a64b55. Accessed 28 Dec. 2021.

[117] "How Exercise Might Help with Acne." *Acne.org*, 16 Aug. 2021, www.acne.org/how-exercise-might-help-with-acne.html.

[118] "Medicinal Botany." *UDSA U.S. Forest Service*, www.fs.fed.us/wildflowers/ethnobotany/ medicinal/index.shtml. Accessed 28 Dec. 2021.

[119] "Frequently Asked Questions on FSMA." *U.S. Food and Drug Administration*, 4 Dec. 2020, www.fda.gov/food/food-safety-modernization-act-fsma/frequently-asked-questions-fsma.

[120] Chiang, Chun-Pin et al. "Anemia, hematinic deficiencies, hyperhomocysteinemia, and serum gastric parietal cell antibody positivity in 884 patients with burning mouth syndrome." *Journal of the Formosan Medical Association = Taiwan yi zhi* vol. 119,4 (2020): 813-820.

[121] Institute of Medicine (US) Food and Nutrition Board. Dietary Reference Intakes: A Risk Assessment Model for Establishing Upper Intake Levels for Nutrients. Washington (DC): National Academies Press (US); 1998. What are Dietary Reference Intakes? Available from: https://www.ncbi.nlm.nih.gov/books/NBK45182/.

[122] Glynis, Ablon. "A Double-blind, Placebo-controlled Study Evaluating the Efficacy of an Oral Supplement in Women with Self-perceived Thinning Hair." *The Journal of clinical and aesthetic dermatology* vol. 5,11 (2012): 28-34.

[123] Patel, Deepa P et al. "A Review of the Use of Biotin for Hair Loss." *Skin appendage disorders* vol. 3,3 (2017): 166-169.

[124] Mock, Donald M. "Biotin: From Nutrition to Therapeutics." *The Journal of nutrition* vol. 147,8 (2017): 1487-1492.

[125] Küry, Sébastien et al. "Clinical utility gene card for: Biotinidase deficiency-update 2015." *European journal of human genetics : EJHG* vol. 24,7 (2016).

[126] Srinivasan, Padmanabhan et al. "Chronic alcohol exposure inhibits biotin uptake by pancreatic acinar cells: possible involvement of epigenetic mechanisms." *American journal of physiology. Gastrointestinal and liver physiology* vol. 307,9 (2014): G941-9.

[127] Donnenfeld, Mathilde et al. "Prospective association between dietary folate intake and skin cancer risk: results from the Supplémentation en Vitamines et Minéraux Antioxydants cohort." *The American journal of clinical nutrition* vol. 102,2 (2015): 471-8.

[128] Kang, Dezhi et al. "Vitamin B12 modulates the transcriptome of the skin microbiota in acne pathogenesis." *Science translational medicine* vol. 7,293 (2015): 293ra103.

[129] Weeks, Benjamin S, and Pedro P Perez. "Absorption rates and free radical scavenging values of vitamin C-lipid metabolites in human lymphoblastic cells." *Medical science monitor : international medical journal of experimental and clinical research* vol. 13,10 (2007): BR205-10.

[130] Michalak, Monika et al. "Bioactive Compounds for Skin Health: A Review." *Nutrients* vol. 13,1 203. 12 Jan. 2021.

[131] Vivarelli, Fabio et al. "Co-carcinogenic effects of vitamin E in prostate." *Scientific reports* vol. 9,1 11636. 12 Aug. 2019.

[132] Heo, Huijin et al. "Protective Activity and Underlying Mechanism of Ginseng Seeds against UVB-Induced Damage in Human Fibroblasts." *Antioxidants (Basel, Switzerland)* vol. 10,3 403. 8 Mar. 2021.

[133] Pierpaoli, Elisa et al. "Supplementation with tocotrienols from Bixa orellana improves the in vivo efficacy of daptomycin against methicillin-resistant Staphylococcus aureus in a mouse model of infected wound." *Phytomedicine: international journal of phytotherapy and phytopharmacology* vol. 36 (2017): 50-53.

[134] Pereira, Gabriela Garrastazu et al. "Polymeric films loaded with vitamin E and aloe vera for topical application in the treatment of burn wounds." *BioMed research international* vol. 2014 (2014): 641590.

[135] Harris, E D et al. "Copper and the synthesis of elastin and collagen." *Ciba Foundation symposium* vol. 79 (1980): 163-82.

[136] Pickart, Loren et al. "GHK Peptide as a Natural Modulator of Multiple Cellular Pathways in Skin Regeneration." *BioMed research international* vol. 2015 (2015): 648108.

[137] Proksch, Ehrhardt et al. "Bathing in a magnesium-rich Dead Sea salt solution improves skin barrier function, enhances skin hydration, and reduces inflammation in atopic dry skin." *International journal of dermatology* vol. 44,2 (2005): 151-7.

[138] Koppes, Sjors A et al. "Efficacy of a Cream Containing Ceramides and Magnesium in the Treatment of Mild to Moderate Atopic Dermatitis: A Randomized, Double-blind, Emollient- and Hydrocortisone-controlled Trial." *Acta dermato-venereologica* vol. 96,7 (2016): 948-953.

[139] Gröber, Uwe et al. "Myth or Reality-Transdermal Magnesium?" *Nutrients* vol. 9,8 813. 28 Jul. 2017.

[140] Niskar, Amanda S et al. "Serum selenium levels in the US population: Third National Health and Nutrition Examination Survey, 1988-1994." *Biological trace element research* vol. 91,1 (2003): 1-10.

[141] Podgórska, Aleksandra et al. "Acne Vulgaris and Intake of Selected Dietary Nutrients-A Summary of Information." *Healthcare (Basel, Switzerland)* vol. 9,6 668. 3 Jun. 2021.

[142] Ozuguz, Pinar et al. "Evaluation of serum vitamins A and E and zinc levels according to the severity of acne vulgaris." *Cutaneous and ocular toxicology* vol. 33,2 (2014): 99-102.

[143] Araújo, Lidiane Advincula de et al. "Use of silicon for skin and hair care: an approach of chemical forms available and efficacy." *Anais brasileiros de dermatologia* vol. 91,3 (2016): 331-5.

[144] Wickett, R R et al. "Effect of oral intake of choline-stabilized orthosilicic acid on hair tensile strength and morphology in women with fine hair." *Archives of dermatological research* vol. 299,10 (2007): 499-505.

[145] "Astaxanthins - an Overview | ScienceDirect Topics." *ScienceDirect*, www.sciencedirect.com/topics/engineering/astaxanthins. Accessed 28 Dec. 2021.

[146] Shibaguchi, Tsubasa et al. "Effect of long-term dietary astaxanthin intake on sarcopenia." *Japanese Journal of Physical Fitness and Sports Medicine* vol. 57,5 (2008): 541-552.

[147] Eisenhauer, Bronwyn et al. "Lutein and Zeaxanthin-Food Sources, Bioavailability and Dietary Variety in Age-Related Macular Degeneration Protection." *Nutrients* vol. 9,2 120. 9 Feb. 2017.

[148] Michalak, Monika et al. "Bioactive Compounds for Skin Health: A Review." *Nutrients* vol. 13,1 203. 12 Jan. 2021.

[149] Juturu, Vijaya et al. "Overall skin tone and skin-lightening-improving effects with oral supplementation of lutein and zeaxanthin isomers: a double-blind, placebo-controlled clinical trial." *Clinical, cosmetic and investigational dermatology* vol. 9 325-332. 7 Oct. 2016.

[150] Palombo, P et al. "Beneficial long-term effects of combined oral/topical antioxidant treatment with the carotenoids lutein and zeaxanthin on human skin: a double-blind, placebo-controlled study." *Skin pharmacology and physiology* vol. 20,4 (2007): 199-210.

[151] Lim, Hyeon-Ji et al. "Inhibitory Effect of Quercetin on Propionibacterium acnes-induced Skin Inflammation." *International immunopharmacology* vol. 96 (2021): 107557.

[152] Galiniak, Sabina et al. "Health benefits of resveratrol administration." *Acta biochimica Polonica* vol. 66,1 (2019): 13-21. doi:10.18388/abp.2018_2749.

[153] Boo, Yong Chool. "Human Skin Lightening Efficacy of Resveratrol and Its Analogs: From in Vitro Studies to Cosmetic Applications." *Antioxidants (Basel, Switzerland)* vol. 8,9 332. 22 Aug. 2019.

[154] Gasparrini, Massimiliano et al. "Strawberry-Based Cosmetic Formulations Protect Human Dermal Fibroblasts against UVA-Induced Damage." *Nutrients* vol. 9,6 605. 14 Jun. 2017.

[155] Pastor-Maldonado, Carmen J et al. "Coenzyme Q_{10}: Novel Formulations and Medical Trends." *International journal of molecular sciences* vol. 21,22 8432. 10 Nov. 2020.

[156] Vollono, Laura et al. "Potential of Curcumin in Skin Disorders." *Nutrients* vol. 11,9 2169. 10 Sep. 2019.

[157] Basharat, Shahnai et al. "Capsaicin: Plants of the Genus Capsicum and Positive Effect of Oriental Spice on Skin Health." *Skin pharmacology and physiology* vol. 33,6 (2020): 331-341.

[158] Kubota, Yoshiki et al. "Novel nanocapsule of α-lipoic acid reveals pigmentation improvement: α-Lipoic acid stimulates the proliferation and differentiation of keratinocyte in murine skin by topical application." *Experimental dermatology* vol. 28 Suppl 1 (2019): 55-63.

[159] Braun, Tara L et al. "A review of N-acetylcysteine in the treatment of grooming disorders." *International journal of dermatology* vol. 58,4 (2019): 502-510.

[160] Curfman, Gregory. "Omega-3 Fatty Acids and Atrial Fibrillation." *JAMA* vol. 325,11 (2021): 1063.

[161] Jayachandran, Muthukumaran et al. "A Critical Review on Health Promoting Benefits of Edible Mushrooms through Gut Microbiota." *International journal of molecular sciences* vol. 18,9 1934. 8 Sep. 2017.

[162] Muszyńska, Bożena et al. "Anti-inflammatory properties of edible mushrooms: A review." *Food chemistry* vol. 243 (2018): 373-381.

[163] Hetland, Geir et al. "Antitumor, Anti-Inflammatory and Antiallergic Effects of *Agaricus blazei* Mushroom Extract and the Related Medicinal Basidiomycetes Mushrooms, *Hericium erinaceus* and *Grifolafrondosa*: A Review of Preclinical and Clinical Studies." *Nutrients* vol. 12,5 1339. 8 May. 2020.

[164] Xu, Xiaofei et al. "Lentinula edodes-derived polysaccharide rejuvenates mice in terms of immune responses and gut microbiota." *Food & function* vol. 6,8 (2015): 2653-63.

[165] Yun, Jong Seok et al. "Inonotus obliquus protects against oxidative stress-induced apoptosis and premature senescence." *Molecules and cells* vol. 31,5 (2011): 423-9.

[166] Hirakawa, S. et al. "Dietary rice bran extract improves TEWL of whole body." *Japanese Pharmacology & Theraoeutics* vol. 41(11): 1051-9.

[167] Gaby, Alan R. "Intravenous nutrient therapy: the "Myers' cocktail"." *Alternative medicine review: a journal of clinical therapeutic* vol. 7,5 (2002): 389-403.

[168] Watanabe, Fumiko et al. "Skin-whitening and skin-condition-improving effects of topical oxidized glutathione: a double-blind and placebo-controlled clinical trial in healthy women." *Clinical, cosmetic and investigational dermatology* vol. 7 267-74. 17 Oct. 2014.

[169] Juhasz, Margit L W, and Melissa K Levin. "The role of systemic treatments for skin lightening." *Journal of cosmetic dermatology* vol. 17,6 (2018): 1144-1157.

[170] Massudi, Hassina et al. "Age-associated changes in oxidative stress and NAD+ metabolism in human tissue." *PloS one* vol. 7,7 (2012): e42357.

[171] Graham, Delyth et al. "Mitochondria-targeted antioxidant MitoQ10 improves endothelial function and attenuates cardiac hypertrophy." *Hypertension (Dallas, Tex.: 1979)* vol. 54,2 (2009): 322-8.

[172] Lieberman, Harris R et al. "Tryptophan Intake in the US Adult Population Is Not Related to Liver or Kidney Function but Is Associated with Depression and Sleep Outcomes." *The Journal of nutrition* vol. 146,12 (2016): 2609S-2615S.

[173] Wang, Dongming et al. "Tryptophan for the sleeping disorder and mental symptom of new-type drug dependence: A randomized, double-blind, placebo-controlled trial." *Medicine* vol. 95,28 (2016): e4135.

[174] Martin, Cresent B et al. "Prescription Drug Use in the United States, 2015-2016." *NCHS data brief*, 334 (2019): 1-8.

[175] Goodarzi, Azadeh et al. "The potential of probiotics for treating acne vulgaris: A review of literature on acne and microbiota." *Dermatologic therapy* vol. 33,3 (2020): e13279.

[176] Lee, Young Bok et al. "Potential Role of the Microbiome in Acne: A Comprehensive Review." *Journal of clinical medicine* vol. 8,7 987. 7 Jul. 2019.

[177] Kober, Mary-Margaret, and Whitney P Bowe. "The effect of probiotics on immune regulation, acne, and photoaging." *International journal of women's dermatology* vol. 1,2 85-89. 6 Apr. 2015.

[178] "How Many Women Buy Skincare Products or Beauty Products Every Year or Every Month or Every Quarter? How Often Do the Buy Beauty or Skincare Products, and How Much Do They Typically Spend per Year on Beauty or Skincare Products? | Wonder." *Wonder*, 27 Apr. 2017, askwonder.com/research/women-buy-skincare-products-beauty-every-year-month-quarter-often-buy-beauty-fe8qyav8v.

[179] "Testimony of Scott Faber, Senior Vice President for Government Affairs, Environmental Working Group." *U.S. Senate Committee on Health, Education, Labor & Pensions*, 22 Sept. 2016, www.help.senate.gov/imo/media/doc/Faber.pdf.

[180] "Sun Protection Factor (SPF)." *U.S. Food and Drug Administration*, 14 July 2017, www.fda.gov/about-fda/center-drug-evaluation-and-research-cder/sun-protection-factor-spf.

[181] Yarosh, Daniel B et al. "Six critical questions for DNA repair enzymes in skincare products: a review in dialog." *Clinical, cosmetic and investigational dermatology* vol. 12 617-624. 29 Aug. 2019.

[182] Luze, Hanna et al. "DNA repair enzymes in sunscreens and their impact on photoageing-A systematic review." *Photodermatology, photoimmunology & photomedicine* vol. 36,6 (2020): 424-432.

[183] Shunatona, Brooke. "Everything You've Ever Wanted to Know About Ceramides." *Byrdie*, 27 Aug. 2021, www.byrdie.com/ceramides-4693671.

[184] Wang, Zhen et al. "Aging-associated alterations in epidermal function and their clinical significance." *Aging* vol. 12,6 (2020): 5551-5565.

[185] Pinnell, S R et al. "Topical L-ascorbic acid: percutaneous absorption studies." *Dermatologic surgery: official publication for American Society for Dermatologic Surgery [et al.]* vol. 27,2 (2001): 137-42.

[186] Pullar, Juliet M et al. "The Roles of Vitamin C in Skin Health." *Nutrients* vol. 9,8 866. 12 Aug. 2017.

[187] Henning, Susanne M et al. "Bioavailability and antioxidant effect of epigallocatechin gallate administered in purified form versus as green tea extract in healthy individuals." *The Journal of nutritional biochemistry* vol. 16,10 (2005): 610-6.

[188] Katiyar, S K et al. "Green tea polyphenol (-)-epigallocatechin-3-gallate treatment of human skin inhibits ultraviolet radiation-induced oxidative stress." *Carcinogenesis* vol. 22,2 (2001): 287-94.

[189] Vayalil, Praveen K et al. "Green tea polyphenols prevent ultraviolet light-induced oxidative damage and matrix metalloproteinases expression in mouse skin." *The Journal of investigative dermatology* vol. 122,6 (2004): 1480-7.

[190] Walocko, Frances M et al. "The role of nicotinamide in acne treatment." *Dermatologic therapy* vol. 30,5 (2017): 10.1111/dth.12481.

[191] Rolfe, Heidi M. "A review of nicotinamide: treatment of skin diseases and potential side effects." *Journal of cosmetic dermatology* vol. 13,4 (2014): 324-8.

[192] Wohlrab, Johannes, and Daniela Kreft. "Niacinamide - mechanisms of action and its topical use in dermatology." *Skin pharmacology and physiology* vol. 27,6 (2014): 311-5.

[193] Schwarcz, Joe. "Reservations About Resveratrol." *Office for Science and Society*, 14 Jan. 2021, www.mcgill.ca/oss/article/critical-thinking-health-general-science/reservations-about-resveratrol.

[194] Widgerow, Alan D et al. "Extracellular Matrix Modulation: Optimizing Skin Care and Rejuvenation Procedures." *Journal of drugs in dermatology: JDD* vol. 15,4 Suppl (2016): s63-71.

[195] Gallo, Richard L et al. "The Potential Role of Topically Applied Heparan Sulfate in the Treatment of Photodamage." *Journal of drugs in dermatology: JDD* vol. 14,7 (2015): 669-74.

[196] Taofiq, Oludemi et al. "Mushrooms extracts and compounds in cosmetics, cosmeceuticals and nutricosmetics—A review." *Industrial Crops and Products* vol. 90,15 (2016): 38-48.

[197] Kalaras, Michael D et al. "Mushrooms: A rich source of the antioxidants ergothioneine and glutathione." *Food chemistry* vol. 233 (2017): 429-433.

[198] Vetvicka, Vaclav et al. "Beta Glucan: Supplement or Drug? From Laboratory to Clinical Trials." *Molecules (Basel, Switzerland)* vol. 24,7 1251. 30 Mar. 2019.

[199] Nakai, Hiroko et al. "Lactobacillus plantarum L-137 upregulates hyaluronic acid production in epidermal cells and fibroblasts in mice." *Microbiology and immunology* vol. 63,9 (2019): 367-378.

[200] Edgar, James R. "Q&A: What are exosomes, exactly?." *BMC biology* vol. 14 46. 13 Jun. 2016.

[201] "Consumer Alert on Regenerative Medicine Products Including Stem Cells and Exosomes." *U.S. Food and Drug Administration*, 22 July 1955, www.fda.gov/vaccines-blood-biologics/consumers-biologics/consumer-alert-regenerative-medicine-products-including-stem-cells-and-exosomes.

[202] Avci, Pinar et al. "Low-level laser (light) therapy (LLLT) in skin: stimulating, healing, restoring." *Seminars in cutaneous medicine and surgery* vol. 32,1 (2013): 41-52.

[203] "Something Happened That Forever Changed My Perspective on Dermal Fillers...." *Victorian Cosmetic Institute*, 18 June 2020, www.thevictoriancosmeticinstitute.com.au/2020/06/something-happened-that-forever-changed-my-perspective-on-dermal-fillers.

[204] Loghem, Jani Van et al. "Calcium hydroxylapatite: over a decade of clinical experience." *The Journal of clinical and aesthetic dermatology* vol. 8,1 (2015): 38-49.

[205] Yutskovskaya, Yana Alexandrovna, and Evgeniya Alexandrovna Kogan. "Improved Neocollagenesis and Skin Mechanical Properties After Injection of Diluted Calcium Hydroxylapatite in the Neck and Décolletage: A Pilot Study." *Journal of drugs in dermatology: JDD* vol. 16,1 (2017): 68-74.

[206] de Almeida, Ada Trindade et al. "Consensus Recommendations for the Use of Hyperdiluted Calcium Hydroxyapatite (Radiesse) as a Face and Body Biostimulatory Agent." *Plastic and reconstructive surgery. Global open* vol. 7,3 e2160. 14 Mar. 2019.

[207] Ronan, Stephen J et al. "Histologic Characterization of Polymethylmethacrylate Dermal Filler Biostimulatory Properties in Human Skin." *Dermatologic surgery: official publication for American Society for Dermatologic Surgery [et al.]* vol. 45,12 (2019): 1580-1584.

[208] Schoenberg, Elizabeth et al. "Platelet-rich plasma for facial rejuvenation: An early examination." *Clinics in dermatology* vol. 38,2 (2020): 251-253.

[209] Peng, Grace Lee. "Platelet-Rich Plasma for Skin Rejuvenation: Facts, Fiction, and Pearls for Practice." *Facial plastic surgery clinics of North America* vol. 27,3 (2019): 405-411.

[210] Maisel-Campbell, Amanda L et al. "A systematic review of the safety and effectiveness of platelet-rich plasma (PRP) for skin aging." *Archives of dermatological research* vol. 312,5 (2020): 301-315.

[211] "Guidance for Industry: Converting Units of Measure for Folate, Niacin, and Vitamins A, D, and E on the Nutrition and Supplement Facts Labels | FDA." U.S. Food and Drug Administration, www.fda.gov/media/129863. Accessed 14 Jan. 2022.

[212] Mithieux, Suzanne M, and Anthony S Weiss. "Design of an elastin-layered dermal regeneration template." *Acta biomaterialia* vol. 52 (2017): 33-40.

[213] "Guidance for Industry: Converting Units of Measure for Folate, Niacin, and Vitamins A, D, and E on the Nutrition and Supplement Facts Labels | FDA." U.S. Food and Drug Administration, www.fda.gov/media/129863. Accessed 14 Jan. 2022.

[214] "UPDATE: The FDA Warns That Biotin May Interfere with Lab Tests: FDA Safety Communication." U.S. Food & Drug Administration, 5 Nov. 2019, www.fda.gov/medical-devices/safety-communications/update-fda-warns-biotin-may-interfere-lab-tests-fda-safety-communication.

[215] Katzman, Brooke M et al. "Prevalence of biotin supplement usage in outpatients and plasma biotin concentrations in patients presenting to the emergency department." *Clinical biochemistry* vol. 60 (2018): 11-16.

[216] Kim, Y-I. "Folate: a magic bullet or a double edged sword for colorectal cancer prevention?" *Gut* vol. 55,10 (2006): 1387-9.

[217] Butler, Christopher C et al. "Oral vitamin B12 versus intramuscular vitamin B12 for vitamin B12 deficiency: a systematic review of randomized controlled trials." *Family practice* vol. 23,3 (2006): 279-85.

[218] "Water Soluble Vitamins." Centers for Disease Control and Prevention, https://www.cdc.gov/nutritionreport/pdf/Water.pdf. Accessed 14 Jan. 2022.

[219] Miller, Edgar R 3rd et al. "Meta-analysis: high-dosage vitamin E supplementation may increase all-cause mortality." *Annals of internal medicine* vol. 142,1 (2005): 37-46.

[220] Ranade, V V, and J C Somberg. "Bioavailability and pharmacokinetics of magnesium after administration of magnesium salts to humans." *American journal of therapeutics* vol. 8,5 (2001): 345-57.

[221] Department of Health and Human Services (US), Department of Agriculture (US) 2015–2020 dietary guidelines for Americans. 8th ed. December 2015 [cited 2021 Feb 22] http://health.gov/dietaryguidelines/2015/guidelines.

[222] Niskar, Amanda S et al. "Serum selenium levels in the US population: Third National Health and Nutrition Examination Survey, 1988-1994." *Biological trace element research* vol. 91,1 (2003): 1-10.

[223] Gene Food. "Genetics and Nutrition Guide." *Gene Food*, www.mygenefood.com/genes. Accessed 28 Dec. 2021.

INDEX

23andMe, 94, 98

A
Aarts, Tom, 142
ablative fractional resurfacing, 217
Ablon, Glynis, 8, 192, 193, 195, 206, 212
ACE Inhibitors, 184
achlorhydria, 46
acne, 38, 39, 41, 52, 53, 54, 55, 56, 75, 83, 86, 89, 90, 111, 112, 113, 115, 117, 120, 128, 131, 132, 133, 141, 154, 162, 164, 179, 184, 186, 193, 198, 199, 204
ADIPOQ gene, 95
advanced glycation end products. See AGEs
AeroGarden, 50
Aethern, 168, 181, 187
AG1, 175
AGEs, 30, 32, 99, 102, 103, 127, 169, 258
Aguilera, Shino Bay, 192, 197, 200
Alastin, 206
ALDH2 gene, 95
All Day Masque Serum, 209
Allergy Research Group, 140
alopecia, 118
alpha hydroxy acids, 197
alpha-lipoic acid, 125, 169
AlphaRet, 200
Alzheimer's disease, 58, 59, 95
American Nutrition Association, 235
American River Nutrition, 140
amino acids, 48, 125
Amino L40, 182

aminoLIFE, 125, 182, 187
amylase, 46
anaphylaxis, 15, 39
Ancestry, 94
Angostura, 47
AnteAGE MD, 119
antibiotics, 184
Apex Energetics, 140
APOA5 gene, 106, 257
APOE4 gene, 95
AquaBiome Fish Oil + Meriva Curcumin, 170
arginine, 125
Arterosil, 181
artificial sweeteners, 37, 83
ascorbic acid. See vitamin C
ashwagandha, 56, 116, 120, 182, 183
astaxanthin, 167, 181, 204
Athletic Greens, 175
atopic dermatitis, 86, 162, 169
autoimmune inflammatory skin, 82
autophagy, 21, 43, 57, 58, 59, 129
Avalon Organics, 198
Avène, 211
Ayurvedic remedies, 85

B
B vitamins, 72, 117, 125, 138, 184
Bacillus coagulans, 208
Badreshia-Bansal, Sonia, 8, 192, 194, 203
Bansal, Vivek, 8
barrier function, 20, 89, 162, 174, 186, 197
barrier protection, 81, 90, 141, 196

BB Primer Broad Spectrum SPF 50+, 195
BCM01 gene, 96
BCO1 gene, 104, 251, 257
Behm, Victoria Yunez, 8
Bellafill, 224
Belotero, 222
Bend Beauty, 181
Berkeley Life Nitric Oxide Support, 175
Best Rest Formula, 182
beta glucans, 173
beta-carotene, 55, 66, 104, 155, 181, 245, 257
BHRT. See Bioidentical Hormone Replacement Therapy
Bifidobacterium, 73, 86, 186, 208
Bioidentical Hormone Replacement Therapy (BHRT), 114
Biological Essentials, 168
BiomeFx, 76, 77
Bionap, 180
biostimulant fillers, 222
biostimulants, 217, 223, 224
biostimulation, 215
Biotics Research, 140
biotin, 151, 243
Bland, Jeffrey, 7, 107
Bodemer, Apple, 192, 193, 198
Bongiorno, Peter, 7
bovine colostrum, 84
BRAF gene, 100
brain-gut-skin axis., 83
Bredesen, Dale, 7, 58
Bryan, Nathan, 175
burning tongue, 145
Bush, Corrine, 8
butyric acid, 74

C

calcium, 160, 246, 252, 257
caloric restriction, 59
candida overgrowth, 76
candidiasis. See candida overgrowth
cannabis, 209
capsaicin, 169
Capsiatra, 169
cardiovascular disease, 57
Carnahan, Jill, 7, 210
carnitine, 126, 154
carotenoids, 65, 168
CD36 gene, 96
CDKN2A gene, 100
CE Ferulic, 202, 203
Celiac disease, 42, 82
cellulase, 46
ceramides, 68, 174, 197
Certified Clinical Nutritionist (CCN), 234
Certified Good Manufacturing Practices (cGMP), 138
Certified Nutrition Specialist (CNS), 234
Certified Personalized Nutrition Practitioner (CPN-P), 235
Cetaphil, 198
cGMP. See certified good manufacturing practices
Chaga, 174
Chan, Gavin, 223
Chilukuri, Suneel, 8, 192, 195, 198, 200, 206
Chiuchiarelli, Jackie, 8
ChromaDex, 177
chrononutrition, 15
citrulline, 125
Clinical Redness Corrector by SkinCeuticals, 204
Coenzyme-Q10, 126, 169, 182
Cohen, Steven, 225
collagen, 19, 23, 32, 33, 43, 55, 62, 66, 67, 75, 99, 100, 102, 112, 114, 121, 122, 141, 154, 156, 161, 163, 171, 172, 173, 180, 181, 196, 201, 202, 206, 217, 220, 224, 225, 226, 227, 228, 255, 256

collagen peptide supplements, 172
collagen peptides, 171
collagen production, 55, 66, 112, 152, 154, 161, 164, 165, 198, 210
collagen remodeling, 215
Color Science All Calm SPF 50, 204
ColorScience, 195
Colostrum-LD, 84, 180
commitment gap, 231
copper, 160, 161, 168, 252, 253, 255
cortisol, 78, 112, 113, 117, 120, 132, 162, 183
COVID-19, 23, 29, 49, 90, 105, 141, 269
Craven, Julia, 8
curcumin, 169, 170, 187, 259
Curél, 198
CYP1A2 gene, 95, 96
CYP2R1 gene, 105, 257
Cyspera, 211

D

dark chocolate, 56
Davis, Isabella, 7
Day, Doris, 8, 11, 192, 209
Dayan, Steven, 8
delayed response reactions, 39
Dermala, 75
Designs for Health, 85, 140, 158, 183
DHT. See dihydrotestosterone
DHT blockers, 120, 122
dietary antioxidants, 63
DigestGold, 47, 187
digestive bitters, 47
dihydrotestosterone, 118
diminished antioxidant capacity, 98
DIND. See drug-induced nutrient depletion
DNA methylation, 108
DNAfit, 110
DNI. See drug-nutrient interaction
Douglas Laboratories, 141, 183

Dover, Jeffrey, 181
Draelos, Zoey, 181
drug-induced nutrient depletion (DIND), 183
drug-nutrient interaction (DNI), 183
DSHEA Act, 141
dysbiosis, 71

E

eczema, 14, 39, 41, 82, 90, 113, 128, 152, 174, 179
elastin, 33, 43, 55, 62, 99, 102, 112, 114, 141, 161, 201, 202, 206, 224, 225, 228, 255
elastogenesis, 226
elimination diet, 40, 42, 56
El-Sohemy, Ahmed, 96, 97, 98
EltaMD, 195
Emepelle, 204
Emerson Ecologics, 140
EMSculpt, 219
emulsifiers, 36, 37, 56
enhancing the skin barrier, 197
Environmental Working Group, 16, 193, 269
    The Clean Fifteen, 51
    The Dirty Dozen, 51
Enzyme Science, 141
Enzymedica, 8, 47, 142, 159, 170, 187, 240
epidermis, 43, 87, 156, 157, 160, 196, 197, 201, 202, 207, 218
epigallocatechin gallate, 204
epigenetic skin tests, 108
epigenetics, 95, 108, 110
Epionce, 196, 210
essential fatty acids, 33, 53, 170
Estee Lauder Revitalizing Supreme+, 196
Estimated Average Requirements (EAR), 35
estrogen, 111, 112, 115, 117, 184, 204

ethanolamines, 193
Etzel, Kendra, 7
Evans, Joel, 7
Everlywell, 41, 146, 232
exercise, 21, 85, 110, 125, 127, 128, 129, 131, 132, 133, 177
extracellular matrix, 43, 197, 201, 205
Eye Shield, 168

F
fake foods, 36
farmers market(s), 51, 69, 177, 179
Fasano, Alessio, 81
fat-soluble vitamins, 151, 155, 180
fiber, 20, 36, 54, 68, 74, 75, 86, 137, 162, 173, 186
finasteride, 118, 119
fissured tongue, 144
Fitzpatrick scale, 219
Fitzpatrick, Richard, 8, 205
folate, 96, 103, 151, 152, 243, 258
folate deficiency, 103
food allergies, 15, 38, 39, 40
Food and Drug Administration (FDA), 138, 194, 244
food intolerances, 38, 39
food poisoning. See gut-based infections
food sensitivities, 15, 38, 40, 41, 80, 110, 231
food sensitivity testing, 41
Forum Health, LLC, 140
Fractional Treatment, 216
Fraxel laser, 216
free radicals. See reactive oxygen species
Frieling, Gretchen, 210
Fullscript, 140
FUT2 gene, 96
FX Chocolate, 56

G
Gaby, Alan, 176
GAGs. See glycosaminoglycans
Gallo, Richard, 207
GammaCore, 78
Garden of Life, 76, 142
Garden of Life Skin+, 76
GC gene, 96, 105, 257
genetic variants, 94, 97, 98, 100, 109, 123
Genopalate, 110
geographic tongue, 143
Gersh, Felice, 7
GI problems, 179
Gilberg-Lenz, Suzanne, 7
Gladd, Jeff, 185
GLO1 gene, 102, 103, 258
glucomannan. See konjac root
GLUT2 gene, 96, 102, 103
glutamine, 85
glutathione, 162, 173, 175, 176, 182, 208
glycated collagen, 20, 32
glycation, 19, 30, 32, 102, 187
glycemic index, 51, 52, 83
glycemic load, 52
glycosaminoglycans, 201
glyphosate, 16, 50, 83
Grain Brain, 82
green tea extract, 204
grooming disorders, 170
growth factors, 205
GSTT1 gene, 67, 104, 257
gut bacteria, 20, 54, 68, 74, 76, 78, 128, 174
gut microbiome, 14, 34, 36, 37, 59, 71, 72, 74, 75, 78, 79, 83, 87, 89, 117, 128, 173, 175
gut-based infections, 46
gut-brain-skin axis, 15, 20, 51, 53, 57, 68, 71, 74, 82, 128, 129

H
HA. See hyaluronic acid
HA Intensifier Serum, 197
hair loss in men, 118

hair loss in women, 120
hair regrowth & needles, 119
hair restoration, 118, 120, 224
Hanaway, Patrick, 7
health consequences of sugar, 52
heart rate variability (HRV), 129
Heilus No.1 Emerge-K, 121
Henry, Michelle, 8
heparan sulfate, 207
hereditary fructose intolerance, 40
Hernandez, Claudia, 8
Heyman, Andrew, 7
hirsutism, 112, 115
HKL-137 Probiotic, 210
Hodzic, Indira, 8
hormone imbalance, 111, 115
hormone replacement, 112, 114, 122, 184
HRV. See heart rate variability
Hu: Get Back to Human, 56
Hughes, Robert John, 8, 285
HUM Skin Squad Pre+Probiotic, 75
HumanN, 175
hyaluronic acid, 62, 161, 170, 171, 180, 181, 196, 197, 222
hydrochloric acid, 46, 153
hydrodermabrasion, 215
Hydropeach, 180
Hyman, Mark, 7, 54
hypochlorhydria, 46

I
IgA antibodies, 39, 84
IgE antibodies, 39, 40, 146
IgG antibodies, 39, 40, 41, 84
IgM antibodies, 39, 84
Immune Max Immuno-Biotic Defense Mints, 209
inflammaging, 19, 33
inflammation, chronic, 124
inflammatory bowel disease (IBD), 37, 250, 254
inflammatory-related skin conditions, 37, 38, 57, 128
Institute for Functional Medicine (IFM), 23, 143
insufficient sleep, 129, 177
insulin resistance, 15, 38, 52, 53, 54
integrative aesthetics, 236
Integrative Therapeutics, 141
Intellishade Clear-Clear, 195
Intense Pulsed Light, 218
intermittent fasting, 15, 57, 59
intestinal permeability, 41, 71, 85, 128
intrinsic factor, 46
ionizing radiation, 63, 101
IRF4, 100, 101, 102, 257
irritable bowel syndrome (IBS), 39
ISDIN Eryfotona Actinica, 195
isotretinoin, 201
IV drips, 154, 176

J
Jacome, Enrique, 7
Jankowski, Bob, 8
January AI, 52
Jogi, Reena, 8, 120
Juvéderm, 222

K
Kamin, Henry, 18
Keaney, Terrence, 8, 118
Keller, Alex, 7
KetoFLEX 12/3, 58, 59
Klaire Labs, 141
konjac root, 75, 86
Krasovsky, Jorge, 8

L
laboratory testing, 145
Labskin, 89
Lactobacillus, 73, 75, 86, 186, 208
lactose intolerance, 40, 47, 252
LaFlore, 208
L-ascorbic acid. See vitamin C

LaValle, James, 7
LC fat transfer, 225
Le Beau, Michelle, 7, 8
leaky gut, 20, 71
leaky gut syndrome, 42
leaky skin, 20, 80
Let's Get Checked, 146, 232
L-glutamine. See glutamine
Li, Huiying, 89
LightStim, 218
Lion's mane, 173
lipase, 46
Lipman, Frank, 7
LipoCalm, 183
Liposomal Zen, 183
Lipski, Liz, 7
LLLT. See Low-level Light Therapy
loss of skin elasticity, 98
Low Dog, Tieraona, 7
Low-level Light Therapy (LLLT), 218
lutein, 55, 66, 168, 181, 259
lycopene, 55, 66, 76, 104, 168, 180
Lycored, 169
Lytera Pigment Correcting Serum, 211

M

magnesium, 117, 126, 145, 161, 162, 246, 253, 258
MC1R gene, 100, 258
McCoy, JD, 236
MCM6 gene, 95
Mediterranean diet, 19, 53
MegaFood, 142
MegaSporeBiotic, 85
melasma, 195, 211
Melatonik, 200
Melatonin PR, 183
Menoloscino, Mark, 7
menopause, 111, 112, 113, 114, 115, 120
metabolic disease, 37

MetaCell Renewal B3 by Skin Ceuticals, 204
Metagenics, 140
Metformin, 184
Microbiome Labs, 75, 84, 85
microdermabrasion, 215
microneedling, 119, 216, 217, 218, 224
micronutrient deficiencies, 249
micronutrient excessive intake, 249
Minich, Deanna, 54
Minoxidil, 119
mitochondria, 21, 43, 56, 57, 101, 102, 123, 124, 126, 127, 129, 149, 154, 177, 218
mitochondrial dysfunction, 124
MitoQ, 126, 182, 187
MMP1 gene, 99, 102, 258
MTHFR gene, 96, 103, 104, 249, 258
mushrooms, 116, 157, 161, 173, 174, 177, 183, 208
My Toolbox Genomics, 110
Myer's cocktail, 176
Myoceram, 174, 180

N

N-Acetylcysteine, 170
NAD+, 126, 177
native antioxidants, 63
Neo40, 175, 181
NeuroCalm, 183
Neurohacker Collective, 183
neurotransmitters, 48, 72, 78, 161
Neutrogena, 211
New Amsterdam Genomics, 97
New Chapter, 142
Nia 24 Intensive Recovery Complex, 204
niacinamide, 204
nitric oxide, 175
non-ablative laser treatment, 216
non-celiac gluten sensitivity (NCGS), 42

Nourish Max vitamin C, B, E and ferulic serum, 203
Now Foods, 142
NQO1 gene, 101, 102, 123, 258
Nutrafol, 121
nutrigenetics, 95
nutrigenomic testing, 20
Nutrigenomix, 98, 102, 109
Nutrisense, 52
nutritional deficiencies, identifying, 143
nutritional genomics, 95, 98, 257

O

obesity, 30, 37, 52, 53, 57, 125
Olay Regenerist, 211
Om Mushroom Superfood, 174
omega-3s, 53, 54, 170
omega-6s, 34, 54, 170
organic farming, 34
Origins, 208
Ornish, Dean, 108
OrthoMolecular Products, 140
orthosilicic acid. See silicon
oxidative damage, 30, 102, 163, 191, 244

P

P. acnes. See Propionibacterium acnes
parabens, 16, 89, 193
Patel, Hetal, 7, 58
PCA Skin, 200
PCOS. See polycystic ovary syndrome
Pegan diet, 54
Pellecome, 113
perimenopause, 111, 114, 117, 121
Perlmutter, David, 7, 82
personalized nutrition, 14
pescatarianism, 48
pesticide drift, 34, 51
photoaging, 66, 86, 100, 124, 157, 161, 195, 258

phthalates, 16, 89, 193
Physician-branded topicals, 209
phytochemicals. See phytonutrients
phytonutrients, 20, 54, 61, 62, 63, 65, 68, 69, 167, 179
pigmentation, 14, 20, 100, 124, 156, 161, 169, 252, 257, 258
pigmented spots, 100, 101
PIH. See post inflammatory hyperpigmentation
Pinnell, Sheldon, 201
plant-based foods, 34, 36, 47, 48, 68, 69, 108, 133, 163, 164
platelet rich plasma (PRP), 119, 217, 224
pollution exposure, 124
polycystic ovary syndrome, 112
polyhydrox acids, 197
polyphenols, 62, 63, 169, 173, 181, 204
Polypodium leucotomos, 61
Pomanox, 180
post inflammatory hyperpigmentation (PIH), 219
potassium, 160, 162, 163, 253, 254
prebiotics, 74, 75
Precisione Medicine Clinic, 84
premature ovarian insufficiency, 111
ProBioSpore, 85
probiotics, 75, 174, 187, 207
Prochaska, James, 229
progesterone, 112, 117, 119
Pro-Nox, 221
Propecia, 118
propionate, 74, 75
Propionibacterium acnes, 88, 101, 154
protease, 46
Proton Pump Inhibitors, 184
provitamin A, 66, 155, 251
PRP. See platelet rich plasma
psoriasis, 52, 82, 83, 103, 131, 132, 144, 152, 153, 169, 179, 198, 199, 258

psychodermatology, 129
Pure Encapsulations, 140, 182
PureWay-C, 154
Pycnogenol, 208

Q
QET, 198
Qualia Life, 177, 187
Qualia Night Sleep Aid, 183
Qualia Skin, 180
Quercetin, 169
Quest Laboratories, 145
QuestAssureD, 145
Quicksilver Scientific, 140, 159, 177, 182, 183
Qunol MegaCoQ10 Ubiquinol, 182

R
Radiesse, 223
radiofrequency, 216, 218, 219
Rainbow Light, 142
randomized clinical trial, 141
RDAs for skin health vitamins & minerals, 243
reactive oxygen species (ROS), 62, 124, 157, 195
Recommended Dietary Allowance (RDA), 34, 49, 150
Red Orange Complex, 180
Reed, Dana, 8
ReFissa 0.05%, 200
Regenacol Skin Inside, 180, 187
Registered Dietitian (RD), 234
Renuva, 225
Replenix, 197
Restylane, 222
resveratrol, 169, 204
ReSync, 187
Resync Recovery Blend, 175
Retin-A, 198
retinal, 155
retinoic acid, 104, 119, 155

retinoids, 155, 196, 197, 198, 199, 200
retinols, 194, 199
Revanesse, 222
revolumization, 222
Revox 7, 206
RHA, 222
Robertson, Lori, 8, 214, 222, 224
Rootine, 110
ROS. See reactive oxygen species
rosacea, 14, 38, 69, 90, 113, 115, 131, 174, 208
Ross, E. Victor, 8, 220
Roundup. See glyphosate

S
Saccharomyces boulardii, 85
SAD. See Standard American Diet
Saxena, Shilpa, 140
SBI. See serum-derived bovine immunoglobulin
scleroderma, 82
Sculptra, 224
seborrheic keratoses, 101
selenium, 116, 160, 163, 164, 181, 184, 254
Sensenbrenner, Scott, 8
Senté, 207, 240
SereneSkin, 75, 186
serotonin, 72, 73, 183
serum-derived bovine immunoglobulin (SBI), 84
Shiitake, 174
short-chain fatty acids, 74
SIBO. See small intestinal bacterial overgrowth
SIFO. See small intestinal fungal overgrowth
Silberman, Adam, 7, 41
silicon, 165
Sinclair, David, 204
Singh, Marvin, 7, 84
single nucleotide polymorphisms (SNPs), 94

Sjogren syndrome, 144
skin aging, 12, 53, 60, 63, 98, 99, 100, 108, 109, 127, 218
skin diseases, 98, 169
skin inflammation, 52, 55, 67, 154, 164, 169
skin, inside, 17, 20
skin microbiome, 15, 83, 86, 87, 88, 89, 90, 207, 208
skin, outside, 17, 20
skin rashes, 39, 164, 251
Skin Trust Club, 89
skin turnover, 43, 197, 198
Skinade, 181
skinbetter science, 195, 200
SkinCeuticals, 132, 197, 202, 203, 204
skin-healthy diet, 127
SkinMedica, 197, 203, 205
SLC30A3 gene, 106, 258
small intestinal bacterial overgrowth (SIBO), 76
small intestinal fungal overgrowth (SIFO), 76
Smith, Ryan, 109
smoking, 31, 63, 66, 100, 102, 116, 124, 127, 244
smooth tongue, 144
SNPs. See single nucleotide polymorphisms
SOD2 gene, 101, 102, 123, 259
solar lentigines, 101
Sovereign Laboratories, 84, 140, 240
Soyier Skin Collection, 210
Spadr, 196
SPF. See Sun Protection Factor
spore-based probiotics, 85
Stages of Change. See Transtheoretical Model
Standard American Diet (SAD), 18, 29, 168
Standard Process, 141
statins, 184

Stephenson, Stacie, 7
Stone, Michael, 143
Streptococcus Thermopolis, 208
Stroka, Mike, 8
Sun Genomics, 76
Sun Protection Factor (SPF), 194
sunbetter SHEER SPF 56 Sunscreen Stick with Titanium Dioxide, 195
sunblock, 61, 194
Sunforgettable Total Protection Brush-On Shield, 195
sunscreen. See sunblock
superoxide, 101, 258, 259
SUPPLEMEANT to Be, 75
supplements for mitochondrial energy production, 181
supplements that build the microbiome, 186
supplements to help with sleep, 182
supplements to compensate for genetic-related insufficiencies, 185
supplements to counter drug-nutrient depletions, 183
supplements to help regulate insulin resistance/glycation, 187
supplements to protect skin, 180
supplements to support immunity, 185
Swidan, Sahar, 119, 210

T
Tan, Barrie, 158
Tannic CF serum, 203
testosterone, 111, 112, 115, 117
TEWL. See transepidermal water loss
Thorne, 141
Thornfeldt, Carl, 210
thyroid hormones, 112, 113
tight junctions, 81
time restricted eating, 15, 57
Titchenal, Jessica, 7

TNS Ceramide Treatment Cream, 197
TNS Recovery Complex, 205
tocotrienols, 158, 187, 252
topical antioxidants, 201
Torkos, Sherry, 7
transepidermal water loss (TEWL), 196
Transtheoretical Model, 230
Trindade, Filomena, 7
tropoelastin. See elastogenesis
Tru Niagen, 177
TruDiagnostic, 109
type 1 diabetes, 81, 82
type 2 diabetes, 16, 38, 52, 53, 57, 78, 83, 123, 184

U

ulcerated tongue, 144
Ulta Lab Test Skin Health Vitamin & Minerals Panel, 145
Ulta Lab Tests, 145
Ultra Firm by AlphaScience, 196
UV Clear Broad-Spectrum SPF 46, 204
UV exposure, 31, 55, 63, 66, 116, 124, 161, 170, 257
UV radiation, 61, 100, 124, 154, 194, 204
UV skin damage, 66, 100

V

VAD. See vitamin A deficiency
vagus nerve, 72, 78, 82
Vampire Facial, 217
Vanicream, 196, 198
veganism, 48, 251, 254
vegetarianism, 48, 254
Vinosource by Caudalie, 204
Viome, 76
Vital Nutrients, 141
vitamin A, 55, 62, 66, 104, 143, 144, 155, 156, 168, 198, 244, 251, 257
vitamin A deficiency, 104

vitamin B12, 46, 143, 144, 145, 153, 154, 249, 250
vitamin B6, 152, 153, 250
vitamin C, 23, 55, 62, 67, 104, 138, 144, 154, 158, 176, 180, 184, 186, 188, 200, 201, 202, 203, 244, 251, 257, 259
Vitamin C + E Complex by SkinMedica, 203
vitamin C deficiency, 104
vitamin D, 23, 105, 110, 116, 137, 156, 157, 185, 251
Vitamin D Council Recommendations, 106
vitamin D deficiency, 105
vitamin E, 106, 157, 158, 164, 168, 169, 185, 202, 203, 245, 251, 257
vitamin E deficiency, 106
vitamin K, 158, 159, 245
vitiligo, 103, 113, 152, 258
Vitreroscilla, 208
Viviscal, 121
Votesse, 121

W

Waldorf, Heidi, 8, 192, 195, 196, 204, 206
water-soluble vitamins, 149, 155
Weleda Skin Food, 198
Wellevate, 140
Wieselman, Brie, 7
wound healing, 55, 60, 66, 85, 124, 156, 157, 159, 164, 165
Wright, David B., 123
wrinkle formation, 53, 98, 124
wrinkle repair, 198

X

Xymogen, 141

Z

Zadeik, Anastasia, 9
Zakaria, Lara, 7
zeaxanthin, 66, 168, 259

zinc, 85, 106, 164, 165, 195, 247, 254, 255, 258
zinc carnosine, 85
zinc deficiency, 106
zinc L-carnosine. See zinc carnosine
zonulin, 81
ZRT Laboratory, 146

ABOUT THE AUTHOR

Mark J. Tager, MD

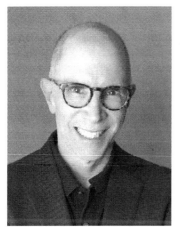

Mark J. Tager, MD is one of the country's leading healthcare communicators. An early pioneer in integrative medicine, he founded the Institute of Preventive Medicine in Portland, Oregon in 1976 where he saw patients for an hour at a time (a rarity!). The Institute featured other holistically oriented practitioners, most of whom also taught classes. Mark taught a popular Monday night yoga class.

He then went on to become Director of Health Promotion for the Northwest Region of Kaiser Permanente where he was responsible for training healthcare professionals to deliver wellness services. While in Oregon, Mark produced a weekly radio show and wrote a wellness column for *The Oregon Journal* and *Seattle Times*. He authored his first of his eleven books in 1977 entitled *Whole Person Healthcare* advocating an integrative approach to medicine. Mark was the producer of an early cable health series sponsored by Bristol Myers Squibb entitled *The Wellness Lifestyle*. After leaving Oregon, he went on to found Great Performance, Inc, a consumer health company that he ran for ten years prior to its acquisition by Times Mirror's Mosby Health division, at the time the leading health science publisher in the United States. He turned over copyright to more than 200 education videos, books, workbooks and posters that he produced.

Mark is currently Chief Enhancement Officer (CEO) of ChangeWell, Inc., where he draws upon his expertise in aesthetic, integrative, and regenerative medicine to helps companies clarify, organize, and disseminate their messages. His consulting clients span the gamut of nutraceutical, cosmeceutical, aesthetic device and clinical laboratory services. He has created a myriad of online training programs for companies directed toward clinicians and/or consumers. He takes complicated concepts and makes them easily understandable. Along with his business partner, Robert John Hughes, he conducts Present*Well*™ Training programs teaching healthcare professionals how to become irresistibly powerful communicators.

Mark was the founding marketing VP for Reliant Technologies where he launched the Fraxel® laser, and then went on to become CMO for Syneron where he launched the Velashape® II. Both devices were among the most successful launches in the field of aesthetics. He also helped launch the cosmeceutical company Senté. He has served as Director of Strategic Initiatives for The American Academy of Anti-Aging Medicine.

Mark actively trains healthcare professionals to improve the care they provide patients. He directs the practice management programs for Miami Cosmetic Surgery & Aesthetic Medicine Conference and serves as an advisor for Informa Markets' THE Aesthetic Show. He has produced a 40-hr, online CME course in Personalized Nutrition for Practitioners for the American Nutrition Association. Mark serves as faculty for Duke Integrative Medicine and consults with numerous specialty nutraceutical companies including Neurohacker Collective, Enzymedica, and Sovereign Laboratories.

In addition to *Feed Your Skin Right: Your Personalized Nutrition Plan for Radiant Beauty*, he has authored or co-authored ten books including *Cash-Pay Healthcare: How to Start, Grow & Perfect Your Business* (with Stewart Gandolf, MBA), and *Enhance Your Presence: The Path to Personal Power, Professional Influence, and Business Success* (with Robert John Hughes). Mark obtained his medical degree from Duke University and trained in Family Practice at the University of Oregon Health Science Center. When not on the road, he hangs his hat in San Diego where he grows impressive tomatoes. He and his wife are visited often by their grown children and first granddaughter.

RECENT BOOKS BY DR. TAGER

AVAILABLE ON

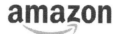

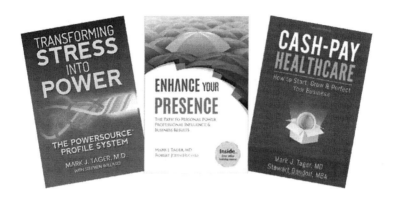

TRANSFORMING STRESS INTO POWER
(Kindle Version Only)

ENHANCE YOUR PRESENCE

CASH-PAY HEALTHCARE

Bonus Offer!
20 Feed Your Skin Right Smoothie Recipes

Get your free copy today!
Scan QR code with a smartphone or visit
DrTagerSmoothies.com

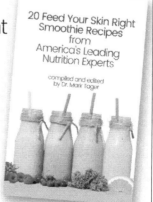

Made in the USA
Middletown, DE
27 January 2025

70195520R00159